More praise for *The Healing Circle*:

"Drs. Rutledge and Walker, an oncologist and a psychologist, have written a wonderfully wide-ranging and compassionate account of adjunctive care for cancer patients, based on their extensive experience conducting healing workshops. Their multi-dimensional approach provides a model of what an extended practice of oncology might ideally embrace."

Alastair J. Cunningham, PhD, Princess Margaret Hospital
Author of *The Healing Journey: Overcoming the Crisis of Cancer*

"I wish I had had this book as a companion piece during my cancer journey years ago. It is an inspirational and intimate source of comfort from the best source of all: people like me, going through what I went through."

Kathy McLaughlin, executive, two-time cancer survivor.

"*The Healing Circle* offers inspirational stories that help you understand the healing process. Its many practical ideas show how you can be more empowered as you open your mind, body and spirit to the wholeness of your life."

Andrew Campbell, retired columnist, writer, business teacher, brain tumour survivor.

The Healing and Cancer Foundation presents

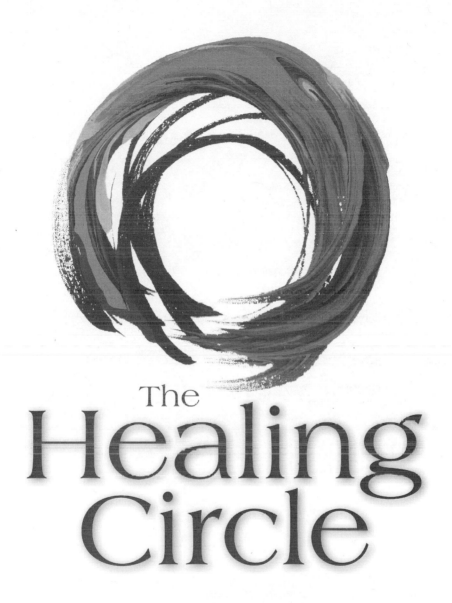

The Healing Circle

Integrating science, wisdom and compassion
in reclaiming wholeness on the cancer journey.

Dr. Rob Rutledge, MD and Timothy Walker, PhD

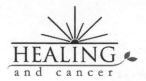

HEALING
and cancer

Editor: Liz Crocker
Design: Kathy Kaulbach, Touchstone Design House
Cover image: Kazuaki Tanahashi, www.brushmind.net

Printed on 100% post-consumer waste paper in Canada.

Health/Cancer/Mind-Body Medicine/Personal Anecdotes/Inspiration

Library and Archives Canada Cataloguing in Publication
Rutledge, Robert, 1965-
    The healing circle : integrating science, wisdom and compassion in
reclaiming wholeness on the cancer journey / Rob Rutledge and Timothy
Walker.

At head of title: The Healing and Cancer Foundation presents.
Includes bibliographical references.
ISBN 978-0-9865465-0-1

1. Cancer--Patients--Care. 2. Cancer--Patients--Rehabilitation.
3. Cancer--Patients--Life skills guides. 4. Healing circles--Canada.
5. Healing. 6. Self-actualization (Psychology). I. Walker, Timothy R., 1956-
II. Healing and Cancer Foundation III. Title.

RC270.8R88 2010   616.99'406   C2010-901367-0

ENVIRONMENTAL BENEFITS STATEMENT

The Healing and Cancer Foundation saved the following
resources by printing the pages of this book on chlorine free
paper made with 100% post-consumer waste.

TREES	WATER	SOLID WASTE	GREENHOUSE GASES
25	**11,515**	**699**	**2,391**
FULLY GROWN	GALLONS	POUNDS	POUNDS

Calculations based on research by Environmental Defense and the Paper Task Force.
Manufactured at Friesens Corporation

DEDICATION

To our mothers who faced cancer with bravery and grace,
And to all those whose lives are touched by cancer,
May they be at peace and free from suffering,
And find fulfillment in reclaiming wholeness.

Table of Contents

Before the Beginning 1

| SECTION I | *EMPOWERING THE BODY* |

Chapter 1   My Healing Journey 7
Chapter 2   Setting an Intention to Heal 12
Chapter 3   What is Healing? 15
Chapter 4   Opening Circle 19
Chapter 5   Andrew: Opening the Door to a New Life 26
Chapter 6   Complete Cancer Care: Part I
             Getting the Best Possible Medical Care 32
Chapter 7   Marie: Riding the Wind and Waves 38
Chapter 8   Complete Cancer Care: Part II
             Empowering the Body 42
Chapter 9   Karen: Accepting and Aspiring 50

| SECTION II | *SETTLING THE MIND* |

Chapter 10   The Power of Mindfulness 57
Chapter 11   Bonnie: Learning to Paddle My Own Kayak 62
Chapter 12   The Raisin Eating Meditation 65
Chapter 13   Coming Home to Your Body 71
Chapter 14   Cathy: Learning to Listen to Myself 77
Chapter 15   Why Meditate? 84
Chapter 16   Kathy: Miracles Can Happen 88
Chapter 17   How to Meditate 95
Chapter 18   My Meditation Practice 102
Chapter 19   Talking about Stress 105
Chapter 20   Practicing the Relaxation Response
             in the Chaos of Life 111
Chapter 21   Pam: Just Being Me 114

SECTION III · *REFRAMING DISTRESSING THOUGHTS*

Chapter 22   "Tell Me About the Place You Come From"... 119

Chapter 23   Reframing "I can't do it"................................ 122

Chapter 24   Geoff: Trading in his Hockey Stick
              for a Walking Stick 128

Chapter 25   Reframing for the Cancer Hero................... 137

Chapter 26   Reframing Distressing Thoughts
              with Kindness and Insight 141

Chapter 27   Jackie: Working Towards Forgiving Myself 148

Chapter 28   Reframing "You're supposed to stay positive"... 152

Chapter 29   Karen: All for the Children 159

Chapter 30   Harry and Ann: Living the Tension
              with Wisdom and Love 164

SECTION IV *RECLAIMING OUR WHOLENESS*

Chapter 31   The Bowl of Loving Kindness Meditation...... 173

Chapter 32   Peter: Letting Anger Come........................... 178

Chapter 33   Embracing Emotions
              with Kindness and Awareness 184

Chapter 34   Jackie: From a Closed Hand to an Open Hand 191

Chapter 35   When Fear is the Teacher 197

Chapter 36   Christine: Heal My Soul or Die Trying 205

Chapter 37   The Story of My Grandmother...................... 212

Chapter 38   Circles Within Circles:
              Spirituality and Wholeness............................. 214

Chapter 39   International Julie Day................................... 223

Chapter 40   "Julie, meet Randy"...................................... 228

Chapter 41   Closing Circle 233

Chapter 42   Continuing the Journey 241

Afterword   My Journey to Healing and Cancer:
              Timothy Walker 244

Acknowledgements 251

Suggested Reading.. 256

Agenda of a "Skills For Healing" Weekend Retreat................. 261

Before the Beginning

"Awaken Heart" was the title of the poster placed just outside the room where physicians review medical charts and dictate letters at our cancer centre. I stopped between seeing patients, curious to absorb these words set in a background of a powder-blue sky. As I read further, my mind seemed to expand and a feeling of calm, mixed with excitement and possibility, came over me. The poster was an advertisement for a stress reduction course offered by Dr. Timothy Walker, a local psychotherapist. Somehow I knew my life was about to change.

At that time, in 1998, I lived in two worlds. Early in my career, as a busy oncologist with a young family, working and teaching at a University hospital, I spent most of my time taking care of people who often shook with fear during their first appointment with me. Through really listening to them, and providing clear information and a treatment plan, I did my best to be a competent and compassionate physician. At medical rounds, in front of my colleagues, I was viewed as a promising physician-scientist.

But my inner world was much richer. I had started to facilitate a weekly cancer support group with the clinic social worker and knew of a space where peace and love seemed to grow, even in turbulent times. I learned healing was possible in a person's life regardless of what was happening on their x-rays. I yearned for a way to marry these two worlds, to empower people by integrating the science of conventional medicine with the wisdom and experience arising in the support groups.

With poster in hand, I immediately set up an appointment with Dr. Walker. I learned Tim had studied mindfulness-based stress reduction with Jon Kabat-Zinn and had been teaching meditation and many other healing techniques for years. Tim drew on the vast teachings of the world's spiritual traditions to present an inspiring message which is simple to understand and universal in appeal.

But what was most striking at our first meeting was his presence. Tim's company brings a feeling of spaciousness, an expanded feeling of compassion and joy. It reminds me of being with some of my pediatric patients who are wise old souls in young bodies. With them, as with Tim, it's as if the rest of the world falls away and time comes to a standstill. Tim taught me how to meditate and, over the last decade, his teachings continue to have a profound effect on my own spiritual growth.

During our first few meetings, we dreamed up a weekend cancer support group called the "Skills for Healing Weekend Retreat" and I began to garner support. The stars aligned. The hospital provided a wooden-floored ballroom free of charge. The Canadian Cancer Society donated $2500 so we could provide lunches and offer the retreat for free. We pinned up and mailed posters far and wide. I hummed with excitement as the big day approached.

The First Retreats

On a Friday evening in 1999, fifty strangers, with all types and stages of cancer, sat in a huge circle of chairs looking anxiously at each other. Tim and I probably appeared just as nervous as we stood up to introduce ourselves. I asked for a volunteer to be the first in the circle to tell a bit about their cancer story and to focus on what was most difficult.

A bright-eyed woman put up her hand and accepted the microphone. With her first few words, the bubble of anxiety surrounding the group disappeared, immediately replaced by a container of compassion. The intense energy of deep caring continued to grow and envelop our group, through our tears and laughter, as we sat, listened, and learned from one another.

By Sunday afternoon, gone were the furrowed brows of Friday evening, and people sat back in their chairs, their bodies relaxed and their faces shining. They exchanged phone numbers and email addresses as they made plans to get together again. I floated out of the ballroom at the end of the retreat, so grateful to have been infused with the love of these wonderful people.

After the first retreat, I figured I had just had a once-in-a-lifetime experience created by bringing together a unique group of old souls. Tim and I organized a second retreat six months later with some trepidation as to what would happen. But when we gathered in the circle, the same loving energy permeated the ballroom and the same magical transformation of forty strangers becoming one community occurred. At the end of the second retreat, an elderly chaplain in attendance commented that, in his thirty years of hospital ministry, he had never experienced the Presence of God as he had during that weekend.

Drawn to Share with Others

Tim and I have gone on to facilitate over 25 retreats in fifteen cities, across Canada and abroad, and the experience has been the same every time. Given the opportunity, it seems we humans naturally and deeply care for one another.

The feedback from the retreats has been tremendous. The high scores on the evaluation forms and follow-up questionnaires are telling, but don't match the stories of people transformed by the retreats. Their willingness to take the next steps on the healing journey fills my heart with joy.

Because Tim and I have witnessed the benefits of teaching this integrated approach to over a thousand people, we now want to share this with a wider audience. We have formed a registered charity called the Healing and Cancer Foundation, hoping to freely offer the teachings to as many people as possible. We've videotaped eight retreats, creating documentaries and educational sets. We've transcribed the interviews and weekend footage of dozens of ordinary yet extraordinary retreat participants. We are continually awed by their lived wisdom and willingness to share the intimate details of their lives.

Reading this Book – Being at a Retreat

This book closely follows the experience of attending a 'Skills for Healing Weekend Retreat.' The chapters more or less alternate between the 'teachings' presented during the weekend and the true stories of people who have attended our program. You will 'listen' to the lectures and talks, learn from the experiential exercises, and sit in on both large and small group discussions. You will 'meet' people who will tell you their stories of how they have worked with the issues being discussed in each section.

The book is divided into four sections, approximating the material presented during the weekend.

Section I, from Friday evening, is called "Empowering the Body." It covers a powerful and integrated approach to a cancer diagnosis, bringing together the best that conventional medicine has to offer with other practical and effective ways to empower yourself physically. Also included is clear advice about how to negotiate the medical system and the science supporting healthy lifestyle choices and the mind–body connection. Following this scientifically-proven advice and practicing the recommended healing skills maximizes the chances of recovery from cancer.

Section II, titled "Settling the Mind", parallels the Saturday morning agenda, and covers mindfulness-based stress reduction and the power of loving kindness. You will learn how to recognize your unique stress reaction and tap into the relaxation response. Tim explains mindfulness and teaches meditation in a way that is simple yet profound. Practising the skills taught here is invaluable in unleashing your body's innate healing potential.

Section III, "Reframing Distressing Thoughts", covers the material taught on the Saturday afternoon of a retreat. The content is a unique combination of modern psychology, mindfulness and loving-kindness. Using multiple real-life examples, we teach how to develop a different perspective of your most difficult situations by drawing on your innate wisdom and kindness. Learning the skill of 'reframing' can have a transformative effect on how you feel about your life.

Section IV, "Reclaiming our Wholeness", offers the experience of a Sunday at the retreat. During this time we introduce the concept that looking at your fears directly and embracing 'negative' emotions can open the possibility of healing your life at a deeper level. Recognizing that your wholeness already exists, we present ways to nurture your inner light on the spiritual path.

I'm excited to offer this book to you because it includes and goes beyond my perspective as an oncologist and presents a practical and integrated approach to the cancer diagnosis. This book focuses not only on physical healing, but also healing that occurs on the psychological and spiritual levels, and your capacity to transform the cancer journey into a journey of the spirit. This book is grounded in love – love for self, love for others, and love for life itself. With mindfulness you can cultivate the energy of loving-kindness to weave love and meaning right into the fabric of your life.

Perhaps, most importantly, I want to share with you the inspiring true stories of many of the retreat participants who have touched me so deeply. These ordinary yet remarkable people have integrated the philosophy of the weekend's teachings into their lives, and demonstrate such courage and resilience through their struggles and triumphs. Each story is different, yet there are universal themes that go beyond the personal stories into the realm of possibility – releasing healing energies that can profoundly affect every aspect of your life.

Section I

Empowering the Body

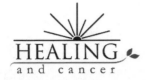

HEALING *and cancer*

Friday Evening • Empowering the Body

In this section of the book, you will sit in the healing circle with fifty strangers as they experience the opening exercises of a 'Skills for Healing Weekend Retreat'. The evening includes hearing stories of some remarkable people and a lecture entitled 'Complete Cancer Care' which outlines a practical and effective approach to a cancer diagnosis.

Integrating conventional medical care with healthy lifestyle habits and wisdom-based healing techniques provides the best chance of healing and recovery from cancer. Through empowering yourself physically, developing the skill of mindfulness, and embracing an attitude of pro-activity and loving-kindness, you will begin to see how wisdom and self-care can manifest in the healing of your body.

To view a seven minute documentary about Andrew (the subject of chapter 5) visit the 'video' link at www.HealingandCancer.org

CHAPTER 1

My Healing Journey

We love because it's the only true adventure.
Niki Giovanni

Friday evening. *Rob introduces himself to the group by telling the story of how he was inspired to become an oncologist and to run cancer support groups.*

When I was a medical student, I didn't know what type of doctor I wanted to be. While psychiatry and working with people with addictions were interesting, what I really wanted to understand was how people cope with the stresses we all face. Medical school catered to my inclination to look at the world as a scientist but I felt there was more to life – something was beginning to awaken in me.

One day as I was browsing in the library, a book seemed to fall off the shelf into my hands. As I stood there, looking at this book, an inner electrical charge surged through me telling me to pay close attention. The book was called "Love, Medicine and Miracles" written by Dr. Bernie Siegel, a cancer surgeon from a prestigious medical school. Bernie was the type of physician who wanted to understand the human side of the cancer experience and was a pioneer in cancer support groups. He felt called to share the wisdom he had gained from his 'exceptional' patients, the ones who seemed to recover quickly from their treatments, whose tumours shrunk faster than expected, who lived longer than all expectations or who even defied the odds of being cured.

Bernie emphasized that his exceptional patients found meaning in their cancer experience and ways to express their love for the people in their lives and for life itself. The stories of ordinary people, showing great courage and strength in their cancer journey, touched me deeply. I remember crying as I read on the subway. From that point on I knew, more than anything, I wanted to be a cancer doctor and to run support groups for those dealing with the disease.

At the end of medical school I learned Dr. Siegel was offering a cancer weekend program for people affected by cancer, followed by a two-day seminar for professionals who wanted to learn more about support groups. We were instructed to read several books including "I Ching", a classic Chinese spiritual text, and a book edited by Ram Dass called "How Can I Help?". It was as if I had been travelling through the desert for years and suddenly discovered water. I couldn't wait to go.

At the weekend program, about 180 people affected by cancer gathered into what looked like a high-school auditorium. I sat in the front row like a keen medical student, wondering what great words of wisdom Bernie would offer this group. How would he inspire us? What lessons would he teach us?

Bernie appeared plainly dressed and, as he leaned into the microphone on Friday evening, his first words were "Hi, I'm Bernie Siegel. I'd like to start out with each of you telling a little bit of your story." With that, he gestured to a man sitting in the back of the room "You sir, can you start us off?" To my amazement, each person stood up in turn and told a little bit of their story.

I remember a young man there with his mother who had ovarian cancer. He sobbed openly, worrying he would lose her. Most everyone was wiping tears from their eyes. Another woman had brought a dead chicken to the seminar and waved it at the group exclaiming that a sense of humour was critical to recovery – we all laughed along.

Story after story, each person shared from their heart and everyone listened intently. The energy in the room was both peaceful and vibrant, and I felt surrounded by compassion and caring. This was my first experience of the magic of a support group. By the time it was my turn, I told the group I had learned more about the human side of cancer in two short hours than I had in all of medical school.

I returned to Ottawa to start my specialist training in Radiation Oncology with that same attitude of trying to learn from the people I was serving every day. More than just providing the best physical care and treating the whole person, I wanted to know how cancer was affecting their lives and what it really meant to them. I learned that listening to a person's story can be therapeutic, and that being able to provide a space where people can share their scariest thoughts and darkest feelings provides a level of healing in and of itself.

Early on in my career, I attended a spirituality and health conference and, for the second time in my life, I felt like I was coming home. I committed myself to ask my patients about their spirituality in a respectful and non-judgmental way during the initial consultation.

The first patient I saw, on the Monday morning after the conference, was an elderly woman with a highly curable breast cancer. Slumped over in her chair, she seemed shaky and nervous. Being jet-lagged and a bit irritable, I just wanted to get to the end of the consultation so I could reassure her that the treatment would be easy and her chance of cure was high. But I forced myself to ask the question "Are you comfortable talking about your spirituality or religion?"

It was as if an inner light had been turned on in her. She sat up straighter in the chair and leaned forward; her face began to shine. "Oh yes, Doctor!" and she went on to recount how she was looking forward to seeing her deceased husband in Heaven. She told me of waking up on the day of her breast cancer surgery with the feeling that the spirit of her husband was lying in the bed beside her. She had felt a great sense of peace and no longer worried about the surgery that day. The presence began to leave and gave her a reassuring pat on the shoulder in the same way her husband had done in their life together. I was touched by her story, and felt I understood her so much better just by asking a simple question.

Many of my other patients shared their spiritual perspectives with me. Another woman, with an early breast cancer, seemed very relaxed during the initial consultation. She explained she wasn't worried about dying but wanted to survive for her young son. She went on to say she didn't pray to be cured of her cancer. Instead she prayed to God to be given the strength to face whatever arises. I was silenced by the power of this insight and kept thinking about her for days afterwards. Like this wise young woman, so many of my other patients have shared of themselves over the years and I am truly grateful for the opportunity to learn and grow from their wisdom.

The Science of the Body-Mind-Spirit Connection

While I was learning from my patients, I was also reviewing the scientific literature to understand what people needed to do to heal from their cancer. Over fifteen years ago, when I first began this investigation, the mainstream scientific community didn't seem interested in health promotion. But in the last few years, science has been showing that simple effective health habits like exercise, a healthy diet, sleep, and relaxation techniques can make a tremendous difference in a person's health, and even in the chance of recovery from cancer.

Science has also been proving the connection between body, mind and spirit. It was fascinating to read about the hundreds of published case reports of people who have undergone spontaneous remission from their cancer. In support of what Bernie Siegel wrote about in "Love, Medicine and Miracles", these remarkable survivors possess certain attitudes and characteristics.

I learned they tap into their innate healing potential by living an authentic, autonomous, and peaceful life filled with purpose and love. They have a deep belief in their body's ability to heal and yet don't worry about future outcomes. They no longer view recurrence of their cancer or even death as a failure and instead put their energy into the things they can control. They listen to their own intuition and the feedback of their body in creating and following a recovery program. They release any sense of guilt about fully loving and supporting themselves. And they also reconnect with their sense of community and reclaim the joy that comes from being of service to others. In healing themselves, they facilitate healing in their loved ones.

I began to share these teachings at public talks and organized a weekly support group for people affected by a cancer diagnosis. (The full story of meeting Dr. Timothy Walker and how we created the 'Skills for Healing Weekend Retreats' is captured in the introductory chapter of this book.)

My Passion to Share

As I stand up in front of a group at the start of every retreat, I feel so grateful to each and every one of the participants for being there, and sharing their stories with me. I know I'm living the dream of a young medical student from twenty years ago. I love this work and feel that I have been buoyed along on my own spiritual journey by these ordinary yet remarkable people.

In the weeks and months preceding each retreat, I set the intention to be a compassionate and wise facilitator, and to be a clear conduit to the profound insights and perspectives I've learned from my patients and participants over the years. I also pray for each and every one of the attendees. I pray that they may gain knowledge and insight, that they may find strength and happiness, and that they may find healing in a way that is just right for them whether it be in body, mind or spirit.

May this also be so for you.

CHAPTER 2

Setting an Intention to Heal

For me, prayer is a surge of the heart
It is a simple look toward heaven
It is a cry of recognition and love
embracing both trial and joy.
St. Therese of Lisieux

After telling his story, Rob asks the participants to join him in a short visualization in which they 'set an intention' for themselves during the retreat. In the same way, you can set an intention for yourself as you begin reading this book.

To set an intention, you first need to drop into a peaceful and receptive state of mind. As you let go of worrying about the future by grounding yourself in the present moment, you are opening to a power much bigger than yourself. From here, you give rise to an aspiration for yourself, to see yourself working towards exactly what is right for you.

You can set an intention in more than one way. You can aspire for a change in your physical health. For example, your intention might be "May I recover from this cancer", or "May I be strong, healthy and flexible." Alternatively, you might set an intention for psychological or spiritual well-being, such as "May I be peaceful, wise and loving in my interactions with others."

The power of setting an intention is that it focuses your energy on a desired state of being. Instead of being pulled this way and that by all the distractions in your world, you focus and draw on the conscious and even more powerful subconscious forces in your psyche. As you drop more and more into the space of intention and align yourself with your deepest purpose, you become more receptive to the opportunities for healing the universe will provide.

However, setting an intention for the future is not just wishful or magical thinking. It changes your perception and physiology in the present. You empower yourself 'in the now'. And then, after you set your intention, you let go of grasping for a particular outcome in the future.

Please join in setting an intention for yourself as you read the following visualization. This is best done if you sit up straight with your feet flat on the floor and you hands resting in your lap or on your thighs. You might want to have someone read this out for you while you sit.

Setting Your Intention – A Visualization

Start by connecting with the sensations in your body.

Bring your attention to your feet planted firmly on the ground.

Feel the sense of gravity and the weight of your body on the chair – allow yourself to take up this space just as you are.

You can straighten your spine so there's a sense of strength and solidity at the back, and yet feel a soft openness at the front of your chest.

Feel as though the crown of your head is being drawn towards the sky

And relax.

Take a few moments to focus on your breathing. You can ask yourself "How do I know I'm breathing?" ..... watch with curiosity.

Watch your abdomen rise and fall. Or feel the sensations of the air going in and out of your mouth/nose and upper airway. Slow down and be curious.

Now begin to generate a feeling of compassion and peace in the middle of your chest. You might think of a loved one or of a little child or of a time when you felt great love and caring for someone special in your life.

Continue to generate the deep feeling of loving-kindness in your heart. You may think of your heart beginning to warm up, like the element on the stove – beginning to radiate an orange or golden energy of deep love that begins to fill up your whole chest.

Take a few moments to generate these deep feelings of compassion and caring.

Now imagine that you could direct this loving energy towards yourself.

You could direct it towards some physical ailment, or a part of your body that needs healing. Pause and feel it.

You could direct this loving energy towards an emotional or psychological problem. You could say "May I find healing to this issue." Pause again.

You could direct this loving energy to a relationship in your life that needs healing.

Extend this sense of peace and love out to a family member or loved one or someone in your life that needs healing – at the level of body, mind or spirit. Pause and wish this for them with all your heart.

Then direct this golden heart energy to everyone else in the world who has been affected by cancer – both those with the diagnosis and their loved ones.

Now, with this limitless source of compassion, set an intention for yourself and release it into the universe.

CHAPTER 3

What is Healing?

We have what we seek.
It is there all the time, and if we give it time,
it will make itself known to us.
Thomas Merton

Friday evening. *Fifty people sitting in a giant circle are listening attentively at the beginning of the weekend retreat. Most have been given a cancer diagnosis; others are their loved ones. They have traveled from near and far to spend this weekend together. Most have left behind busy lives, others long days spent on a couch. Some arrived early, happy to break the routine of retirement; others rushed in at the last moment from work or family responsibilities.*

Some have been recently diagnosed, fresh out of surgery, their dressings hidden under brightly coloured blouses and sweaters. Others have traveled many arduous miles along the cancer journey. Some are bald or wear wigs and scarves that attest to ongoing chemotherapy. Others look perfectly well. Women and men, young and old, well-attired and casually dressed, all are waiting, a little nervous but excited to begin.

The people sitting in the circle on Friday evening are looking to us as the "experts"– the ones who will teach them how to heal their lives. In fact, the power lies with them. With lifetimes of experience, everyone in this circle has vast resources of wisdom and the potential to transform within themselves. Through their openness, their resolve to empower themselves, and their courage to walk into the unknown, they can discover their own path. They really are the experts in their own lives.

Tim, a therapist and spiritual teacher, honours the group and begins by explaining the meaning of healing:

The word healing comes from the same root word for 'wholeness', 'health' and 'Holiness'. Healing means to move towards wholeness. To heal doesn't necessarily mean to be cured of cancer – although that is always possible. As you heal your life, your physical health can improve dramatically and you can increase your chances of recovery.

Wholeness has to do with reclaiming all aspects of yourself – your body, mind and spirit – and bringing all these parts back together. When you heal you can connect more deeply with everyday life and something bigger than that – something that we might call spirituality. As you move towards wholeness, you begin to experience the depth of who you really are.

We each have tremendous wisdom for healing and transformation but sometimes we don't have time to access it because life is so filled with details. We get caught up in stress and distraction and forget about wholeness and our capacity to heal.

This is why a retreat is a precious opportunity for us. It is a time when we can open up a door within ourselves to see what is there, to let in some fresh ideas and new possibilities. We can briefly step out of the rushing stream of our lives to find an island of peace and stillness, a place for calm reflection.

I believe that the moment we come through that door and enter into this circle of chairs—what I call a healing circle—we are entering into a sacred kind of space and time, a time where we can slow down enough to get to know ourselves more deeply, and a space where we can truly connect with others in a way that is real and satisfying. The healing circle is a space, like a gentle container, where we can practice loving ourselves and reclaim our already existing wholeness. The retreat allows us to uncover that treasure which is the healing power within our own human heart.

Jackie has been listening intensely but doesn't understand the part about "reclaiming her already existing wholeness." She is a 45-year-old mother of three who worked full time as a nurse when she was diagnosed with breast cancer ten months ago. A loving woman who was used to "taking care of everyone else," she bravely marched on through chemotherapy, wearing the smile of optimism for everyone to see.

Now two months off treatments, the suppressed worry and stress, coupled with her physical exhaustion, have left Jackie raw, irritable, and on the verge of tears. As she looks out at the others in the circle, her stomach aches as she thinks about the possibility of recurrence. She worries about how her husband and kids would cope without her and feels that she is a terrible burden on her entire family. As fears play in her mind, she struggles to make her distressing thoughts and painful feelings go away.

Tim continues his introduction by asking the group questions that are also on Jackie's mind: "How can we be whole and yet feel so broken? Where is our wholeness when we are in so much distress? How can we find that deep well of peace when our life appears to be shattered?"

John sits up straighter in his chair when he hears the word "shattered". In the prime of his life, his leukemia has forced him to walk away from an executive position in a software firm. He is frustrated with how weak he is after months of chemotherapy and feels disoriented by the total loss of his identity as a successful businessman and head of a family. Fair-weather friends have disappeared and family conflicts have created awkward silences and emotional distance. He feels that his whole life has been ripped away from him— he feels 'shattered'.

Jackie, John, and many others in the circle have come to the weekend because they want to be cured of their cancer and they want to feel happy again. The retreat offers a simple and effective way to work toward these goals, but at times its approach may seem paradoxical. Participants are asked to be proactive and do the practical things that will maximize their chance of recovery, but they are also asked to suspend their attachment to any specific outcome.

Instead of trying to control what will happen in the future, Tim asks people to focus on what they can do in the present, to find a wellspring of wisdom to guide them in reclaiming the joy of wholeness that was there all along, but may have been hidden under the intensity of striving for a particular result.

The cancer journey, and life in general, contains some degree of suffering. Acknowledging this is an essential step in reclaiming a sense of wholeness. Embracing turbulent emotions has a transformative effect on one's whole being. Most people want to reject their awful feelings, dispelling the energy by acting out or stuffing them down into shadows of the psyche. But deep within these so-called "negative emotions" lies the energy of life and a doorway to profound insight.

For Jackie, John, and the others in the healing circle, the process of reclaiming their already existing wholeness begins by simply showing up, showing up with all their fear, anger, and despair – as well as their courage, fortitude, and wisdom. Tim invites everyone present to bring all of themselves into the healing circle for the weekend—all their awkwardness and self-critical judgments as well as their laughter and joy. Showing up just as they are gives them a real and solid place to begin, a ground of truth from which to start their journey.

Tim continues his talk, saying "Our physical bodies are part of our wholeness, but this is not the whole picture. Our physical experience is nested within our psychological and social realms, and nested in awareness itself. Wholeness and healing are about integration, about bringing all of these parts together— synchronizing our body, mind, and spirit.

"We are shattered yet whole. To struggle with this paradox is itself a process of healing. The loss, sorrow, and pain—and everything that can come with a cancer diagnosis—brings us to a bigger understanding of what it really means to be human. This is what we'll learn on this retreat."

The people in the circle seem to be settling back in their chairs. In a moment of silence a few people turn to their loved ones to whisper, or smile at each other and hold hands. Others look across the circle, curious and somehow uplifted by all the people in the room. Others seem to be looking deep into themselves, as if remembering a sense of wellness. The nervousness in the group is fading, and a sense of possibilities and purpose begins to arise.

CHAPTER 4

Opening Circle

When your fear touches someone's pain,
it becomes pity; when your love touches
someone's pain, it becomes compassion.
Stephen Levine

Friday evening. *Rob facilitates the first group exercise by asking everyone sitting in the large circle to take one or two minutes to introduce themselves by telling a little of their cancer story, what has been most difficult during their journey, and their hopes for the weekend.*

There is an uncomfortable silence when people realize they will be sharing the intimate details of their lives with fifty strangers. Rob asks for a brave volunteer and waits.

Earl raises his hand. He is a small pale man in his sixties with a thin white beard and dark-rimmed glasses. He looks comfortable in his V-neck sweater. His wife is beside him, her arm across his back. Earl's voice is soft, almost hollow, but he is articulate and seems completely at peace with himself. "I was diagnosed with prostate cancer five years ago. I've found myself on the wrong side of the curve every step of the way. I now have metastatic cancer that's gone through the bones and into my internal organs.

"I'm in the middle of the reprieve that comes from the hormone therapy. I'm doing great. I have a little bit of trouble justifying all the special attention I'm getting." He squeezes his wife's hand, then looks brightly out to the others. "But I'm getting used to it." He continues in an even voice, "The biggest problem I have is the effect it has had on Pat"— he taps his wife on the knee, "and the rest of my family. For me, a kind of acceptance came with the diagnosis. But it was painful to see people having to absorb this bad news as it came on to them rather quickly. We thought the cancer was under control, then it shot through the roof."

Earl pauses, then offers his hope for the weekend: "I'm looking for heart connections and more." He raises his eyebrows briefly and smiles gently.

Earl is unlikely to undergo any type of transformation during the weekend. He already rests calmly in a place of deep peace, acceptance, and love for his fellow travellers. He'll bask in the energy of the group, listen closely to their stories, and immerse himself in the group exercises. He'll support others whenever he can, like volunteering to speak first in front of the group. His inner radiance is already a guiding light for others, especially those who have been recently diagnosed. Near the end of his life, this man is very much alive.

Pat is younger than Earl, her dark hair woven evenly with grey. "Pretty much everything Earl said, I can echo. When we found out about the spread to the liver, I had a couple of weeks of crash and burn. I came out of that, but I still go into it every once in a while. Right now I'm struggling with work responsibilities and wanting to spend as much time as I can with Earl. So it's been a real roller coaster. Probably this group would understand that it is both the best time of our lives and the worst time of our lives."

Pat smiles at Earl. "In this weekend, I'm looking for the strength and skills that will take me through the future, no matter what that brings."

Nancy is next. A forty-year-old mother of teenagers, a nurse with a full bright face and brown caring eyes, her voice begins to tremble as she tells her story. She motions to the thin white-haired lady sitting beside her. "I'm here in support of my Mom. Cancer has touched our lives a number of times. My father had metastatic prostate cancer. My mother had breast cancer and now she has peritoneal cancer. Right now, I'm overwhelmed by everything that's happened. My husband has just been diagnosed with Alzheimer's as well." With this she begins to cry quietly. Her mother reaches over and pats her on the shoulder. Nancy tries to continue. "I'm feeling…", but she just continues to cry.

I let out an audible sigh and support her show of emotion. "It's OK to cry. Just stay with it"

People are listening closely and I can sense a feeling of great caring in the room. Nancy finishes with, "I'm hoping to gain strength this weekend for the journey ahead. I want to help the people I work with, and my family."

Nancy's mother takes the microphone. She is a perky and positive person. "The hardest thing for me is the guilt that I have given this difficulty to my three daughters and son. They have all accepted it. And so we are moving on. I am very busy and enjoying life. My chemo is over now. I sailed through that." She runs her hand through her short curly hair, and then says with a laugh, "Now I have curls." She wants to make Nancy feel better.

The group laughs as they continue to waver between touching their own pain and trying to stay positive. Several people already have tears in their eyes and I encourage everyone to share the boxes of tissues found under their chairs.

The next person to speak, a stocky middle-aged French Canadian woman with short hair, rests back easily in her chair. She's confident, outgoing, and willing to express the truth as she sees it. Three years ago she was diagnosed with a rare type of cancer called carcinoid. There's still anger in her voice when she says she was sent away from the emergency room and dismissed by her gynecologists three times before being diagnosed. She admits, "Being angry is one of the things coming up right now. I've had surgery and two bouts of chemo and right now I'm on vacation." She smiles broadly at the group showing the humour that resurfaces through her introduction.

"The worst part is the anger, the stress, the effect on my husband, who is a double amputee. And the uncertainty." She almost cries through her words. "Cancer is a blessing in a way but it's also a curse. I find I can cope well most of the time, but at night I'm having a hard time. I'm glad I'm getting in touch with my feelings because I can use humour as a deflective device."

She finishes by foreshadowing the work we'll do this weekend. "We're going to be looking at things that I've tried not to look at too much. I understand the more you try to control your thinking, the more you become obsessive. So I want to enjoy myself and work with those thoughts in the background."

I thank her and reinforce that we welcome all emotions this weekend, including her anger.

The next woman is in her fifties and has been on treatment for multiple myeloma, an incurable type of blood cancer. Her face is pudgy from years of treatment with steroids. She shares with the group her reaction to being told over a decade ago that she had eighteen months to live. "I waited. And I waited. And waited. And I'm still here. And I'm not going anywhere." She's calm and smiles broadly at the group. "I've learned to accept it and live my life from day to day. I realize the next flu season could take me away." Her manner is light and refreshing. "I just enjoy my life."

Kathryn is a 37-year-old real estate agent. Her smile is infectious, and the group energy instantly lightens. She is quick to express her frustration at having stage three colon cancer. "I had a bowel resection last June which I hated. I really don't like hospitals. I thought I would take a week off after the operation and then go back to work. Ha! Ha!" People recognize that Kathryn is laughing at her own naiveté and laugh along as she giggles.

She continues in a serious voice. "It took me a real long time to recover from that. I couldn't get my energy back. I'm a single mom with three kids and this has devastated me financially. I lost my confidence. I felt I lost my life spirit. I was probably suffering from depression." The group is taken aback by this admission of vulnerability from someone who looks so 'together.'

Kathryn shares that she decided not to take the recommended chemotherapy and seems to be doing well. "My treatment plan is working, so I'm happy about that. But my doctors feel my stress level is in the danger zone, so that's why I'm here. I really need to learn some stress reduction techniques for my healing."

A large walker sits in front of the next woman. She is big and it's obvious from her thin voice she has many health challenges and other difficulties in her life. She lists her struggles one after the other, in sentence after shocking sentence: she suffers from mental illness; she hopes for her own death so she can join Jesus in heaven; she writes about herself as the "despised person." She summarizes her anguish: "It's very hard to live with, and so if I say something unkind to you, I ask for forgiveness. I hope for this weekend that I'll be in contact with Almighty God and that He'll guide me." The group listens attentively. This woman has been totally welcomed.

Maureen is obviously upset, her voice trembling. Five years ago, in her mid-forties, she was treated for kidney cancer and seems to be cured. She feels lucky now. She turns to the good-looking man beside her and begins to tear up. "But my husband was diagnosed with an aggressive brain tumor. I'm a glass half-full type of girl so I want to learn a few skills so I can stay half -full."

Maureen's husband takes the microphone and glances at his wife with a smile. "My name is Frank. I'm sorry I'm a bit shaky" His voice is wavering with emotion. "I had my tumor taken out on Christmas Eve.

"The most difficult issue," he continues very slowly, "is to receive the love all the people are giving me. I'm having a hard time. I've never been a receiver. I've always been a giver." The tears are streaming down his face. There's a long pause and he lets out a big sigh before he says with determination, "I believe in the power of my mind. What I want to get out of the weekend is hope and how to make it work." I sense a feeling of intense compassion building in the air.

Andrea jumps to her feet. She's a big and bubbly woman in her early thirties, doing well after treatment for breast cancer. She explains that a friend bought her a large coffee that afternoon, and, "she didn't order it decaf! I'm just wired here! I've been sitting here almost crying the whole time."

Everyone laughs as the tension is released. Andrea stays on the light side of her journey. Several others are thankful for the reprieve from the emotional intensity. But as the stories come, one after the other, they are naturally drawn to listen with compassion and empathy.

Rick has tears in his eyes as he listens to his wife, who was successfully treated for breast cancer four years ago. He is a hefty man with long wavy hair and a greying goatee. He drives a truck for the postal service and races cars in his spare time. His voice is pitched higher than usual, emotions caught in his throat. "I've been diagnosed with prostate cancer, and it's pretty serious. I'm on hormone treatment now." He wipes away his tears. After a pause, he bursts out crying. "And my mother passed away three weeks ago from a brain tumor.

"I hope to get some skills out of this weekend to help myself and to feel better." Seeing this rugged man cry brings the group into a deep silence and a true appreciation of his pain.

The next woman is on the verge of tears. Rick has provided her an opportunity she has been seeking. She's over the physical effects of her breast cancer, but realizes she has denied her feelings through the whole process. She says, "I really want to get close to my feelings. I want to mourn the loss of my life before cancer."

I look around the room and can see most of the people have a tissue in hand and have released some of their sorrow. With the intensity also comes a lightness, a feeling that there is more space in our hearts.

Ed has a brain tumor, which has come fifteen years after a testicular cancer diagnosis, and he struggles with the uncertainty of the situation. Debbie, Ed's wife, complains that "once you finish with one doctor, they send you off to another one. And they just cut you loose. You're just drifting. They never see you again." She summarizes, "The medical system has been a bit unsupportive."

More and more stories. People speaking from their hearts. Everyone listens with rapt attention. David is the father of Valerie, a beautiful young woman with a brain tumor. Valerie takes the microphone from her father and they glance at each other with love in their eyes. Her tumor appears dormant after surgery, radiation, and chemotherapy, but everyone feels the sadness of a young woman taken away from her imagined future. "My dream was to teach and I was teaching in Japan when this happened. I don't think I'll ever teach again. And I'd like to be a mother, but that's been put on hold too. I hope this weekend leads me to the path where I can start working again." David wraps his arm around his daughter and she collapses into his shoulder. Our hearts are raw. People begin to wonder how long this can go on. We are only halfway through the circle.

Patty has just been diagnosed with breast cancer, and the staging tests show spots on the liver and lungs. "The most difficult thing so far"—her voice turns squeaky, tears streaming down her cheeks—"has been to tell my family. Because it makes them so sad. I wonder what I should have done so this would not have happened. I hope this weekend we can learn to deal with some of those things. Thank you all for sharing with us." I make a note to myself to emphasize in the lecture later that evening that getting cancer was not her fault. But for now we will simply hold her pain.

Wally is Patty's husband. He is a retired executive in his sixties and owns several companies. He has always been a "take charge" type of person. As he watches his wife he wipes the tears from his face. He blows his nose, slumping down, staring at the floor. His body begins to heave, trying to release the deep sobs of sadness. He holds himself in, pushing the tears back as they well up. He takes a deep breath. A few more seconds pass. He takes another long breath. Patty jokes, poking her husband in the shoulder, "...and Wally is my greatest strength."

I wait for the laughter to die down so everyone can hear the seriousness of my voice: "This is strength that you're seeing right now." After a pause I add "Let it come. You have a deep heart."

Wally's voice lilts up and down "It's been very difficult not knowing what the future holds. We are both results-oriented people and we had a life planned. We've done a lot of things together and I don't want it to end." Wally turns, his head lowered towards Patty, and she holds onto him tightly.

People are tiring now. I can hear a shuffling in the chairs. They are asking themselves, "How can I go on? How can I take any more?" People do not yet realize that listening to the last twenty people in the circle will be a spiritual lesson as their hearts will keep opening with compassion.

Jan has lost her creativity. Kathy has had to accept the possibility of dying to facilitate her amazing recovery. Julian is dealing with the cancer by himself. Velma is surprised by her outburst of tears, having held onto the pain for so long—for her son's lymphoma diagnosis five years ago and for her husband's recent brain tumor. Theresa is cured of a lung cancer the doctors said was terminal ten years before. Her journey was "a wonderful experience".

Remarkably, for all the pain, suffering, and tears in the room, so many people keep saying how struck they are by the strength and courage they hear in each others' stories. The circle is generating a powerful feeling of love.

Anne passed the first time around, so she is the last person to speak. Her ovarian cancer came at a stressful time in her life. "I was single, lost my job in a mass layoff, and was about to start my own business when I was diagnosed." Her voice is weak with exasperation. "That was the last straw because I wasn't able to do anything, much less look after myself! I was told, 'We need six more months of your life to give you chemotherapy.' I wasn't sure how I would support myself… much less find the strength I needed.

"For my whole life I was someone who looked after other people. I was strong for people. But now I need to care for myself. I need to rebuild my confidence and my life.

"I focus on the word 'retreat' for this weekend because it takes me away from all the responsibilities I have. I am so grateful to have this time here with you."

After everyone has spoken, I reassure them that the whole weekend will not be as intense as this opening exercise. I encourage them to stay with whatever emotions have come up, listening to so many stories at once.

"Sharing and listening to stories can touch you in many ways. Stories can be inspiring and they can also bring up many different emotions; there is great value in welcoming them all. When you allow yourself to feel sadness, grief and pain, you stretch your heart, opening more space to appreciate the preciousness of life and the joy of living."

CHAPTER 5

Andrew
Opening the Door to a New Life

Andrew was lying on the stretcher outside the operating room, overcome with a profound and inexplicable sense of peace and an inner feeling that everything was going to be fine. It made no sense. At 58, his life as a successful business consultant, newspaper columnist, husband and father had been completely shattered. The operating room nurse interrupted his reflections to confirm his identity. "What's your date of birth?" she asked.

"March 5, 1948," Andrew responded but he added in his own mind that he was also born a second time, just two weeks ago, on Christmas Eve, when he suddenly fell ill. His cancer diagnosis arrived as "a present wrapped in barbed wire". Velma, his loving wife of thirty years, woke up to a violent shaking in the bed. (He joked later, "Not the type of shaking you want to have on your bed.")

Andrew was trapped in a grand mal seizure; he was shaking uncontrollably, gritting his teeth, eyes staring deep into nowhere. Velma called the paramedics. The seizure continued in the ambulance, into the emergency room, shaking the life out of his body. Forty-five minutes later he was sedated. His CAT scan showed a tumor the size of a tangerine in the front of his brain, but the doctors couldn't be sure if it was malignant. Surgery would follow in two weeks.

As his nurse wheeled him into the operating suite, Andrew was still aching from the seizure that ripped his muscles, yet he felt an incredible sense of peace that defied any sense of reasonableness given what was to come. Dr. Bernstein, a renowned neurosurgeon, was about to drill out a large piece of bone, cut through the normal brain tissue, and carefully dissect out as much of this tumor as possible—all while Andrew was awake.

This 'awake-craniotomy', done as a three-hour day-surgery procedure, is used to minimize effects on the normal brain. But even with the cutting-edge technology, Andrew and Velma had been told that he may come out of surgery with his emotions flattened, expressing no joy or sorrow, or so irritable and lacking in insight that he'd blow up uncontrollably— or his mental function may be so compromised he'd 'wake up like a vegetable.' Regardless Andrew relaxed into the table, enveloped in a peace that passed all the understanding that he'd ever known.

Andrew's thoughts were drawn to his 96-year-old mother-in-law. A decade earlier, when Andrew's sense of humour had exceeded her tolerance, she suggested that he should have his brain examined. Now, lying on the stretcher, Andrew mused that "With an elementary school education, she knew the diagnosis long before the 'doctor-guy' with the long list of letters behind his name and fifteen years in university."

Andrew also contemplated his mother-in-law's initial reaction to hearing that he had a brain tumor. "Andrew, you have not been listening to God." He later wrote, "This was quite a remarkable insight which blurted out of her mouth automatically. Perhaps it was a blinding glimpse of the obvious to her; however, to me, that insightful chord struck deep. It was one that I listened to and that still lingers in my mind—often during my daily meditations."

Andrew was willing to peer deeply into any situation, listen to every comment, and investigate it with an open heart and mind. Instead of being angry at his mother-in-law for a thoughtless comment, he thought about what he could learn from her way of thinking.

The surgeon started his saw. It made a terrible grinding sound like a powerful coffee blender. It took Andrew over a year before he was able to go into a coffee shop for fear of this terrible sound.

With his fingers deep in Andrew's brain, the neurosurgeon asked Andrew if he was seeing anything unusual, trying to assess whether Andrew's brain was being irritated by the manipulation. Suddenly, Andrew was pulled upwards and inwards all at once. He saw a beautiful purple/violet flame, an image that mysteriously appeared twice during the operation. He was no longer just in the 21st century; he stretched himself back in time more than two thousand years. The songs of wisdom passed down for generations echoed in his head: "Ezekiel saw a fire a-burning, way in the middle of the air … a fire within a circle of fire a-burning…"

His visions of a spiritual light reminded Andrew of his father-in-law, Arthur. As a young man, Arthur emigrated from Britain, farmed in Northern Ontario, and then served in World War II. Called to the ministry on his return, he brought his wife and three young daughters to Montreal, where he attended McGill University's School of Divinity.

Arthur and his family were dirt poor but happy and thriving until he suddenly contracted meningitis and fell into a deep coma. His fellow divinity students organized an around-the-clock prayer vigil, praying to God to save this inspirational young man. Dr. Wilder Penfield, the pioneering neurosurgeon who first performed awake-craniotomies, the same procedure that Andrew was undergoing, was called in to try to save Arthur's life. Penfield watched as Arthur's body shrivelled, and two weeks later suggested that the family gather to say their last goodbyes.

Meanwhile, Arthur felt angels pulling him to heaven. He felt himself going through a tunnel with a brilliant array of colors that are not seen in this physical world. He felt such a profound sense of peace that he was sorry he had to return to this world. But he understood his time had not come and his work was not done.

The next morning Arthur was sitting up at his bedside eating breakfast. Dr. Penfield was dumfounded and called it a miracle. Arthur went on to serve others in the ministry for 47 years and had an enormous impact on many people. He had a deep love of nature, the earth, the planets, and the stars. He truly wondered about the magnitude of the sun, the sky, and how the universe came together. To him it was more than just idle chatter.

The same forces that hold the stars together and allow the grass to grow were working in Andrew's body as he was wheeled to the recovery room, then in the car ride home later that same evening.

Andrew believes he thought about his father-in-law on the operating table because he was expecting a miracle as had happened to Arthur. His belief that his brain tumor happened for a purpose has not wavered. But the wait for the results and his experience over the next few months clouded over his faith in a bright future. It took two long weeks for the doctors to process the specimen from Andrew's brain. The diagnosis: anaplastic oligodendroglioma, a rare but aggressive tumor affecting about 1 in 10,000 people with a cancer diagnosis. Andrew was completely beside himself when told that without further treatment he had perhaps a year to live.

Fortunately, another test showed that the tumor had a special genetic change (1p19q) that meant Andrew could be offered a new chemotherapy. Andrew is extremely grateful to the medical professionals who provided this state-of-the-art treatment and he quickly agreed to take the chemotherapy every month for a full year. His physical healing had begun.

But, everything in Andrew's life had changed. He could no longer work. His ability to concentrate and think clearly was compromised. Even filling out insurance forms, something that would have been a snap just two months earlier, left him gritting his teeth in frustration. He was on edge, no longer able to hold up the mask of the competent consultant.

As a result of the seizure, he lost his driver's license and was forced to be a passenger, a role he had never played in his previous life. Still agitated from hearing that he might have only a year to live, when he saw his wife make a lane change too quickly, he swore uncontrollably. "For ★!#$★ sake, Velma, what are you doing?" Thankfully, Velma could see how the stress of the situation and the damage to his brain was at the source of his emotional ups and downs. She could easily forgive Andrew the outbursts, for he was also more open emotionally. Velma says she loves Andrew even more the way he is now.

Andrew felt overwhelmed by multiple stressors in his life including sorting out all the issues in his house, the fear of the unknown, his anger, dealing with death, and making medical decisions when given conflicting information. Andrew reflects back on this dark period and says, "Sure I was fine. I slept like a baby…I'd wake up every few hours and cry." He can laugh now, but he acknowledges that it took time to heal from a profound grief.

For months Andrew felt like he was being tossed in waves of emotional turbulence, but at the same time had an overwhelming sense that something much bigger than himself was buoying him up. He was working to be both proactive and willing to surrender, to re-learn how to trust in the journey and to accept his struggles.

His personal mantra throughout his journey has been "Pray as if it is up to God, but act as if it's up to me" and as the poet Anthony Mizzi said, "Every problem offers new possibilities for something wonderful to happen." Andrew is too busy looking at the door opening in front of him to be concerned about the one that has been shut behind.

So while receiving the best that modern Western medicine can deliver, Andrew did everything else he could to maximize his chances of recovery. He attended many counselling sessions, something he would never have considered a year before. He used his 'beginner's mind' to follow his intuitions about what Eastern and other complementary medical approaches could offer. He changed his diet, exercised more, lost weight, allowed himself more sleep, began a daily meditation practice, became a Reiki Master, practiced Qi Gong—whatever made sense and felt right. In some sense he was going with the flow, and listening to God as his mother-in-law had suggested.

Andrew was led to Dr. Alastair Cunningham, an immunologist-turned-psychologist, who himself had undergone a spiritual transformation just before being diagnosed with an aggressive colon cancer. Dr. Cunningham created and ran the Healing Journey program at a university hospital in Toronto since 1980.

A study of Dr. Cunningham's pioneering work showed that people like Andrew, who have been given an incurable diagnosis and who take a proactive and positive approach, often live longer than those who are only mildly interested in integrative care. Some of the study participants who were highly involved in their own healing are alive with no evidence of cancer more than a decade after their physicians expected them to die.

The Healing Journey program introduced Andrew to the concept that cancer cells grow in the body chemistry or 'soup' created by the molecules in the bloodstream and that he could change the soup through his actions and his mind. Andrew wanted to change the ingredients in his life. Many of the things that fit into his old life did not fit his new life, and so he sold his house and car, gave away old furniture, closed his business, and retired. He and Velma moved to a new city where they felt they belonged and began life anew.

Another key teacher on Andrew's journey towards wholeness was Adam, the Dreamhealer. At age sixteen, Adam first gained notoriety when he helped facilitate the miraculous healing of rock star Ronnie Hawkins. Apparently the distant healings and the visualizations Hawkins learned from Adam were critical to his complete recovery from a medically incurable pancreatic cancer.

Andrew had taught a corporate version of visualization to executives in his previous work, but his own healing visualizations were a much more intense experience. He would picture his tumor cells being zapped by lightning bolts and energy packets and then turned into a dusty substance that was expelled in a shower of light. Andrew learned the success of his visualizations depended on fully engaging his emotions in the process. He truly felt he was making changes to the cellular structure of his cells.

Remarkably, from being a highly controlled person who always lived in his head, Andrew feels the cancer diagnosis cracked his emotional shell wide open. A caring comment from a friend will bring tears to his eyes and a frog in his throat as he peers deeply into their eyes and heart.

He wants to dance at hearing happy music and cry with sad music. The aromas and odours that he smells are more distinct. He can smell carrots five feet away and flowers from thirty feet away. The pungent smell of a pig farm in the country is as wildly exciting as car fumes are painful. "Life is so vibrant that it is like when I fell in love with my wonderful wife."

Andrew is incredibly grateful for the opportunity to experience the wholeness of life and is committed to serve others for whatever time he has left. He does not believe it is his time to die yet. He says, "There's still more 'stuff' to do."

How long he will remain on this earth is no longer a concern to Andrew. "I have surrendered with acceptance. It's not my choice of when I come and go. As far as I know, I may have some input and I can do all I can while I'm here. But that final decision is not mine. There was a great relief when I started to accept that."

An entry from his daily journal reads, "As long as the human spirit rises to the challenge of each new day, as long as we pursue worthwhile goals, as long as we strive, suffer, wrestle with our difficulties and endure, and find wonder in the world, we are living our dying with love."

Now, more than three years after his original diagnosis, there appears to be no indication that his tumor will recur. He may 'live his dying with love' for years and years to come.

CHAPTER 6

Complete Cancer Care
Part I - Getting the Best Possible Medical Care

God grant me the serenity to
accept the things I cannot change,
The courage to change the things I can,
And the wisdom to know the difference
Serenity Prayer

Friday evening. *Many of the people in the opening circle are living through the first few weeks and months of a cancer diagnosis and are looking for practical and effective advice about what they can do to maximize their chance of recovery. Drawing on his expertise as a cancer specialist, Rob outlines the approach of combining the best of western medicine with healthy lifestyle habits and wisdom-based complementary healing techniques. In the first part of this lecture, he provides advice on how to get the best care from the medical system by adopting a proactive and loving attitude towards yourself.*

The marriage of scientifically-based treatments and wisdom-based healing practices is called 'integrative medicine'. This integrated approach, also called 'complete cancer care', will give you the best chance of living well after a cancer diagnosis. By empowering yourself at the level of body, mind and spirit you can make a tremendous difference in how you feel, in your general health, and even in your cancer outcome.

Getting great care from the medical system is at the foundation of 'complete cancer care', and is an exercise in paying close attention to what is happening, recognizing the truth for what it is, and taking the appropriate action.

Pay Attention to How You Feel

At different stages in the journey, you'll focus more on some elements of complete care than on others. For instance, gathering information and making the best possible medical decisions will dominate your thinking at the time of diagnosis and early on. Working with the emotional fallout of cancer often peaks near the end of your treatments. Nurturing your spiritual life can happen to various degrees throughout the journey.

There is no 'best way' to approach a cancer diagnosis. Everyone is different both in terms of their personality and in terms of their cancer situation. Therefore, you'll need to engage your rational mind as well as your intuition in working towards a program and strategy tailored to your needs.

Gather Information Mindfully

Carol Shields, the Pulitzer-prize winning author, wrote that being diagnosed with advanced breast cancer was like waking up on a train in the middle of a stormy night in a foreign land where everybody spoke a different language. So, the first essential step in working with the medical system is to understand this language.

What can make this complicated is that most people are highly stressed when they are diagnosed with a life threatening disease, and it's much harder to learn new information when you're stressed. As well, cancer is a complicated disease, everyone's case is unique, each person has their own way of learning optimally, and we all learn at different rates.

Being mindful in this 'foreign land' referred to by Carol Shields allows you to focus your attention on what's happening in the outer world as well as to your inner reaction. As you gather information, you can ask yourself "Do I understand what I'm being told? Is this useful?" and at the same time ask "How does this information or situation make me feel?"

Some people feel driven to get as much information as possible about their cancer, staying up late at night surfing the net for the latest breakthroughs. By way of contrast, there are some people who don't want to know anything and so don't seek out any extra information. In both of these cases, there may be underlying psychological issues. In the first example, the person may be hoping information will give them control over the situation, and in the second case, the person may be in a state of denial. In both cases, being mindful about their feelings could be an important first step to a deeper level of healing.

If at any time you're feeling overwhelmed with the information you're reading, you can recognize those feelings and take steps to change what you're doing. For example, by being mindful, you might realize that obsessing over information is actually depleting you of life energy. You can pay attention to your inner wisdom to do what you need to do. One strategy may be to ask a loved one to gather information for you. Either way, honouring that you have psychological limits, even while being appropriately proactive, is a clear act of kindness towards yourself.

Understand Cancer and its Treatment

Try to understand the basics about cancer: its causes; how it is detected; how it can cause problems; and how it is treated. Learn about your particular case: the type of cancer; if it has spread and, if so, how far it has spread (stage); other factors determining how serious your cancer might or might not be (prognostic factors); and your treatment options. Ask about and consider the risk and benefits of each treatment option, including the option of deciding not to pursue active treatment.

By having a general understanding of cancer and the main concepts of treatment, you'll be better able to understand your cancer doctor and to collaborate in making the best medical decisions together. Don't worry if you don't understand everything at first and don't hesitate to ask for information to be repeated or for time to reflect. Acquiring information and insight is a continuous process as you become more familiar with the details of your case.

Major hospitals and most cancer centres have a librarian that can help you gather information in a way that is easiest for you to absorb and that is specific to your situation. As well, there are many books, pamphlets and hospital websites which provide reliable information. Community-based organizations like the national Cancer Societies offer free information services through their websites or toll-free numbers. They often provide trained information specialists who can also tailor the information to your needs.

Remember that information gathering can be tricky because you can quickly become overwhelmed with too much information. If trying to find good information is tiring, then give yourself a break.

If you decide not to become an expert in your own care, then ask a loved one to play that role. It's helpful to have a second set of ears hear what you are hearing and to have someone else understand what's happening. This person can help you review appointments, and also be ready to advocate for you and with you every step of the way.

Be an Active Participant in Your Own Care

Prepare for your appointments in advance by writing down any questions you have, and bringing copies of test results with you. If possible, bring someone with you to every appointment. Beforehand, decide who will record or remember the information. At the visit be open and honest and, if need be, ask for clarification from your cancer doctor when you're unsure or feel you are receiving conflicting advice.

Another way to empower yourself is to have a copy of your own medical file. Because the medical system is a human institution, and sometimes reports go missing, most physicians appreciate it when you come up with a photocopy of a missing lab test or have summarized the results in a nice graph—this saves everyone valuable time.

I recently had a discussion with one of my breast cancer patients about starting a new hormone pill. I warned her about the possible side effects, including thinning of the bones. I wanted to order a bone density test before I started her on the medication. She reached into her bag and pulled out a binder with her complete medical history. She flipped to the 'bone' section and showed me a normal bone density report from three years before. A quick photocopy, a prescription for her new medication, and we both went away satisfied.

She had obtained a copy of her test results by going to the medical records department of her hospitals and her other physician's office, quoting her legal right for a copy of everything written about her. She updates her file by requesting a copy of every new report.

Remember You are the Most Important Person

Try not to be intimidated by your cancer doctors. Remember the reason for your appointment is to make sure that you're receiving the best possible care. Make sure the session works for you. For example, if your doctor is talking too fast or using overly complex language, speak up. A simple line like, "I'm sorry, I'm feeling a bit overwhelmed. Can you repeat that a bit more slowly?" or "I don't know that word you just used…can you explain it to me?" can put you back in the driver's seat.

It is empowering to understand the facts of the situation. The medical system is meant to deliver the best possible physical care for you. You have a right to understand what's happening in your body and to review the pros and cons of the treatment options with your doctor. You are the most important person in the clinic or hospital room—not your doctor.

You can use the same attitude of pro-activity and self-love in reviewing the appointment afterwards. Do you feel you had all your questions answered? Are you getting conflicting information? Are there any other professionals or services which could help you with the problems you are facing? Do you have a clear understanding of what the care plan is during treatment and in long term follow-up? What are your responsibilities? What can you do to improve your health and chance of recovery?

If you feel your medical team can help you more, then say so, and ask for what you need. If it's answers to questions that you need, call for clarification or ask for an appointment. The cancer centre nurse may be able to address many of these questions and concerns. And, as one of the weekend attendees recommended, 'Squeak gently but persistently.' Ultimately the squeaky wheel gets the grease.

When you advocate for yourself, you send a powerful message to your body and psyche about healing and wholeness. By being proactive and by being fully collaborative with the people on your care team, you can feed the flame of inner confidence, heighten your inherent strength, and invite in the universal capacity to heal.

Become More Comfortable with the Unknown

As you learn about cancer and its treatment, you'll quickly discover that medical science does not have the answers to all the questions about cancer. For instance, why any one person develops cancer while someone else does not is not fully known. Scientists know that certain habits, like smoking, predispose people to cancer, but multiple other factors may also contribute such as genetics, the aging process, other environmental contaminants, an impaired immune system or just plain bad luck. The point is you may never know what caused you to develop cancer.

When you can accept that there are many unknowns in the causes, treatments, and the possible outcomes of cancer, then you can begin to let go of trying to know, for certain, what the future will bring. You can then focus your energy on the things you can control in the present.

For example, you *can* get the best care offered by the medical system and you *can* empower yourself. With a foundation of knowledge and a plan to be a partner in your own care, you can begin to relax and tap into the incredible healing potential of connecting with others, expressing both your fears and your love, and finding meaning and purpose in your journey.

CHAPTER 7

Marie
Riding the Wind and Waves

Marie tossed in bed. Her mind was still churning over yesterday's medical appointment. Her oncologist had told her that her PET Scan showed activity in her sternum and he couldn't tell if her breast cancer had come back — only a year after her diagnosis. Marie then looked up to the two pictures on her bedside table which she had placed there to 'anchor' and guide her healing journey.

The first picture shows her standing on a beach in France. It was taken two years before her breast cancer diagnosis at age 38. As a single woman, Marie had joined a tour visiting the shores of Normandy. The brisk wind and sound of surf invigorated her as she quickly headed to the water's edge to begin a long walk, the waves breaking at her feet.

After some time, an old man who was on the tour offered to take her picture. Marie posed, facing up toward her new friend. Both were unaware that a huge wave was bearing down on her. When it hit, crashing around her body, the wave threw her to the sand, soaking her to the skin. The tour bus would not return until the end of the day and Marie lay wet, shivering, and out of breath.

Pledging to herself to make the most out of the day, she got up, brushed the dirt off her clothes, and began to walk around. Shivering at first, she accepted a jacket from a stranger and then joined her new friends who were climbing the rocks and cliffs, warming herself through the vigorous climb. Before long, she was laughing, enjoying the spectacular views, and by lunchtime was dry enough to sit with her friends and taste the French bread, cheese, and wine.

Marie understands the wave in this story to be her cancer diagnosis and looks to this picture as a reminder that she can choose how to respond to life's difficulties. Trained as a child psychologist, she took a positive and proactive approach to her diagnosis and the months of chemotherapy, mastectomy, radiation, and two reconstructive breast surgeries. She empowered herself with information, drawing on the expertise of the cancer centre librarian, as she prepared for each of her medical visits. She would just smile at her plastic surgeon when he teased her about bringing in a pad of paper with questions.

Marie was also quick to integrate healthy habits into her life like exercise and a healthy diet which had recently been proven to improve breast cancer survival rates. She started taking the stairs instead of the elevator, or would park several blocks from the school where she worked which added a brisk walk to her day.

Her healing program also included mindfulness meditation that she learned from the cancer center's social worker. She learned a 'playful' healing visualization in which she imagined her white blood cells as white beluga whales going into the sand to remove cancer cells.

Although Marie felt empowered by the practical things she was doing to promote her healing, she had to work with the anxiety that she wasn't doing enough. At one point, she struggled with feelings of guilt for not exercising as much as she thought she should. But she learned to reframe these thoughts with a kind and rational response by telling herself she was doing the best she could, focussing on 'baby steps' instead of trying to be perfect.

As Marie cherished her alone time, the individual self-care activities came easily to her, but she worried about her support system. In the years leading up to her diagnosis, in which she had a busy clinical practice and was teaching at the university, her social circle was shrinking and she was feeling less connected to her family. When she found a cyst in her breast that didn't go away, her greatest fear was not of dying but of being alone – single and isolated during her cancer journey.

She remembered working with children with cancer during her training, and being awed by their courage and resilience. Drawing on their inspiration, she deliberately chose to break away from her tendency to withdraw and, instead, to share the news of her diagnosis with all of her friends and family, even reaching out to colleagues at work.

Marie was overwhelmed by the emails, phone calls, and gifts of support. Her mother, who lives in another city, came to live with her. Someone would come to each of her medical appointments to take notes for her.

It was initially intimidating for Marie to even think about joining a support group, but the experience was so positive that she invited these same women to meet in her apartment every month. They would share their lives with each other and laugh over silly things like the time when

Marie described getting a cold scalp when she stuck her bald head in the fridge.

Marie gave each woman a stone that had been smoothed by the waves from the beach near her cottage. The members of the 'stepping stones' group carried these solid reminders of their connection to each other in their purses. Just before Marie was to undergo her second breast surgery, the women gathered in Marie's apartment where they signed her 'stepping stone'. She carried it with her into the operating room and now brings her stone with her everywhere she goes, a reminder that she is connected to the invisible web of her healing community.

When one of the group members suffered a recurrence, Marie stuck with her friend every step of the way, providing rides or meals, or simply listening to her in the last days of her friend's life. This experience was rewarding but also provoked Marie's fears, especially when Marie's PET scan raised the question whether her own cancer had come back. More than ever, she needed to draw on the inspiration from her second healing picture.

This second picture was taken shortly after her treatment finished, when her brother invited her to go sailing. The winds were very strong that day and the boat tilted at a precarious angle as it shot through the water at breakneck speed. Her brother asked her to take the steering wheel. Marie's eyes opened wide as she recounted the scene. "He was yelling at me, 'You can do it—Go! Go! Go!' I was scared but laughed at the same time and stayed at the helm despite my fear. I was able to do it. So that's the way I want my healing journey to be— I want to stay at the helm of my boat even if it's frightening. And I will find some joy and meaning in it. "

Marie smiled to herself as she recalled seeing this picture posted on the fridge door of one of her 'stepping stones' friends. She had sent out invitations to forty close friends and family members to join her in an "End of Chemotherapy / Fortieth Birthday" Party. The idea for this party began during an art therapy exercise at our weekend retreat.

Marie had drawn pictures representing her life in the past, the present, and the future. The picture of her future was a montage of people joyfully gathering in a beautiful building, warmed by a golden sun in the background. Marie felt awkward about the idea of inviting others to such a celebration but a close friend finally persuaded her to send out the invitations.

Everyone showed up. People brought baked goods and told stories about Marie. She reflects "So that was a big event and people really enjoyed it. And at that celebration I gave a talk and showed the drawing I had done at the weekend retreat. I told people how, in a way, cancer had been a gift for me. It sounds strange to say that, but I discovered how strong I was, and how loved I was, and how much support I had in my life. Being alone was not an obstacle. I had so many people in my life.... And I'm trying to have this sense of celebration every day now."

Five years after the questionable PET scan, Marie appears cancer-free and no longer needs to take hormone therapy.

CHAPTER 8

Complete Cancer Care
Part II- Empowering the Body

Anything we do with a whole heart
can be a prayer
David Steindl-Rast

In the first part of the Friday evening lecture, Rob defined Complete Cancer Care as the marriage of conventional medical care with mindfulness and wisdom-based healing attitudes and practices. This second part of the Friday evening lecture focuses on how to empower the body — the essential elements of care for everyone with a cancer diagnosis.

As an oncologist, Rob wants to show this diverse group of people how to be proactive in making lifestyle choices and, paradoxically, to relax more. He wants to offer the participants a simple plan to cover all their bases, so that, with this plan, they can appreciate their own power and let go of searching for a magic bullet somewhere else. Rob believes that with a loving attitude towards one's body and by trusting in one's innate wisdom to guide decisions, people can make a tremendous difference in their physical health and happiness.

Several years ago, I heard a keynote speaker at a lymphoma conference, a top-notch journalist who had undergone bone marrow transplantation which consists of extremely high doses of chemotherapy.

This man, who was very fit before his transplant, was left weak as a kitten in his hospital bed in the days that followed. But he was determined to strengthen his body. Wisely, he began to build himself up in slow increments.

For the first week of his exercise program, he simply pulled himself out of bed and onto a bedside chair. During the second week, he moved the chair across the room, forcing himself to take a few tentative steps each day. By the time he went home, he could walk to his front door in a single go.

And what do you think he was telling himself, subconsciously, during the fourth week, when he made it to the end of his driveway? What was the message to his spirit during the fifth week, when he strolled to the corner of his lot?

He was saying "I want to get strong. I want to be well. I love this body of mine and I'm willing to do what it takes to get better." He was taking his frustrations, anger, and fear and channelling them into a loving act of self-care and healing. At a profound level, his body and mind responded to his message.

General Advice

Being proactive with your health sends a powerful message to your mind and body about healing and wholeness. By adopting the attitude that your body is very precious, you can learn and practice skills and lifestyle choices that facilitate strengthening and healing your body.

Consider the 'body' elements of complete cancer care – exercise, diet, weight, sleep and relaxation. Work on what you consider to be the most important elements first and then incorporate others as you see fit. Trying to follow *all* of the advice provided in this chapter *at the same time* may not be practical and might cause unnecessary stress or guilt.

Just as it is good to be purposeful, it is also good to have some time each week to simply reflect and do nothing. Promoting healing is about balance, and listening to your intuition. Nurturing your body requires that you draw on the wisdom of your body, solid scientific evidence, and a deep sense of love for yourself.

Essential Elements in Complete Cancer Care

1 • *Exercise*: An important element in strengthening your body is to pursue some form of exercise. Even those who are physically weak from treatments or their cancer can benefit from encouraging their body to become stronger by exercising up to and just beyond their comfort zone. For some people, this might be walking around the block and for others it might be much more. Everyone is different in terms of what they can do or where they can start, but exercise is key to maintaining and improving strength, flexibility and energy for life.

Studies are now emerging which show how exercise can improve survival for people with cancer. The scientists believe exercise suppresses the blood levels of hormones and other molecules responsible for cell growth, such as insulin-like growth factor, which appears to increase a cell's ability to divide and cause cancer.

A number of high quality studies show that people who exercise before, and even during, chemotherapy can maintain their energy levels better than those who do not exercise. The training effect of having your body routinely exert itself actually changes how your cells process oxygen and other nutrients. Even your brain functions better after exercise.

One particular study involved people with incurable cancer (most of whom had cancer that had spread to other parts of their bodies) who were taught a simple program of a six-minute walk, sitting to standing knee bends, and an arm reaching/stretching drill. The program took 50 minutes twice a week for six weeks. At the end of those six weeks, the participants reported a real improvement in quality of life, less physical fatigue and shortness of breath. Compared with their pre-program assessments, they were 20 percent faster at getting out of a chair and could reach an average of one inch farther with their hands.

Furthermore, exercise burns off sugars, fats, and other stress reaction by-products; decreases inflammation; and improves your immune function. Interleukon-6, a key chemical in the anti-inflammatory pathway, can increase a hundredfold after exercise and the release of interleukon-6 boosts your ability to fight off infections and probably cancer cells as well.

Exercise strengthens your body physically, allowing you to do more. The benefits to your heart, lungs, blood pressure, bones, and weight can be impressive. Whether your goal is to simply get out and see more of this beautiful world or to exert yourself on a dragon boating team, exercise is very helpful.

The Optimal Exercise Program

Now the question is 'What is the optimal exercise routine for you?' To find out, start by talking to your family doctor. He or she can provide advice or refer you to a physiotherapist who specializes in exercise programs. If you have the means, you can even seek out a personal fitness trainer to work with you on an ongoing basis to enhance all three pillars of your physical health: cardiovascular reserve, strength, and flexibility.

Pursuing your own exercise program can works especially well if you mindfully listen to your body for feedback. One woman who had joined a dragon-boating team noticed that she felt especially happy the day after a strong workout but felt that her energy waned if she booked too many hard workouts in a single week. Science shows that overly intense exercise will suppress the immune system. Allowing the body time to rest and heal is as important, at times, as building muscle or enhancing cardiovascular strength and endurance.

The internet and books are a great source of information about how to slowly and consistently make progress with exercising. Even something as simple as going for a thirty-minute walk three times a week is a reasonable goal; or you can dance to some music at home or use a stationary bike or get into the water. The objective is to have fun and get your heart rate up and feel it pumping blood, and nourishing every cell in your body

Whenever you start exercising, especially if exercising is new for you, there's a critical moment when you may feel uncomfortable and feel like giving up. It's important to know you won't hurt yourself and that encouraging yourself through this threshold is where you start gaining the benefits of exercise. Exercise provides the perfect opportunity to draw on and strengthen your inner fortitude, and develop the capacity to push beyond the first few minutes of exercise when you might feel uneasy and out of breath. This same sense of determination can be applied when you run into psychological discomfort or relationship challenges.

Deciding to exercise as part of a healthful and loving life is not meant to create an extra stressor, something else you need to cram into your schedule. Even doing just a little bit initiates positive change. Your body will continue to change and adapt to what you can do. When you exercise routinely, you'll feel happier and have more energy to do the things you love to do. In addition to strengthening your body, exercise releases endorphins; the hormones that make you feel good. Studies show that people who exercise have improved mood and quality of life, feel more relaxed, sleep better, and enjoy enhanced feelings of independence and self-confidence.

The benefits of exercise appear to be further augmented by following a healthy diet high in fruit and vegetables. A recent trial following women with potentially curable breast cancer showed a 5-7 percent increase in survival at 10 years when women exercised for 30 minutes five times per week and ate 5-10 servings of fruits and vegetables a day compared with other women who did not practice both of these healthy habits. Data suggesting the survival benefits of exercise and diet is also emerging for other types of cancer.

2 • *Follow a healthy diet:* "What you need to do is change the soup." I am referring to a new field of science called Epigenetics which shows that cells are not only driven by their internal genetic code but also by the hormones and other chemicals which bath them. Every cancer cell has to adapt to a unique kind of soup in the body before it can live and grow. Along with following the other healthy lifestyle habits, choosing a healthy diet is an especially powerful way to 'change the soup', improve your overall health and sense of well-being, and is a necessary ingredient in the recovery from cancer.

The science linking diet and cancer is well established. In 2007, the World Cancer Research Fund published a 500-page report entitled *Food, Nutrition, Physical Activity and the Prevention of Cancer: A Global Perspective.* The top 200 cancer prevention scientists from around the world examined why there is a global epidemic of cancer. Their conclusion? Because of access to so much unhealthy food in the last 200 years, our diets have become a major risk factor for cancer.

Although the report focused on *preventing cancer,* the scientists suggested that people who have been given a cancer diagnosis would likely benefit from this same advice about modifying what they eat. The same dietary factors which contribute to developing cancer can potentially cause further changes (mutations) in cancer cells lingering in the body – turning slowly growing cells into cells which could replicate faster and spread. You can 'change the soup' by increasing fruit and vegetable consumption and by ingesting antioxidants which can mop up cancer-causing chemicals. Through a healthy diet, new cancers are less likely to form, and cancer cells which may not be obvious are more likely to remain in a dormant form.

Essentially, these international studies support a diet which includes a complex combination of nutrients to allow your tissues to be healthy or to heal. The reason to avoid extreme diets, eating a balanced diet at each meal instead, is that the micronutrients from one food group support the micronutrients from other food groups in building and repairing tissue. The *Canada Food Guide's* current suggestions are simple and effective:

- Eat several servings of fruits and vegetables daily, including at least one dark green and one orange vegetable

- Choose whole grain products.

- Drink low/no fat milk or fortified soy products (if your body tolerates them).

- For your protein needs, choose meat alternatives frequently, such as beans, lentils, and tofu.

- At least two servings per week of a fish, or another food high in omega-3 fatty acids, is recommended

- An organic plant-based diet, high in fruits and vegetables, with healthy protein supplements, is by far the most life-enhancing choice. Shop around the periphery of the grocery store, staying away from the processed food in the middle aisles. Drink plenty of healthy fluids, especially water, so your overall intake of calories remains relatively low. Flush out your bowel system with a diet high in fibre.

The Optimal Diet for You

No matter what the scientific information is, however, you will still need to adapt your diet to match your body's particular needs.

If you're in the midst of treatment, it's best to get advice from your cancer doctor. As most physicians have limited training in nutrition, you should probably ask your doctor or nurse to refer you to a trained nutritionist. Getting advice from an expert would be especially helpful if your treatment or the cancer is affecting your mouth or digestive tract; is causing diarrhea/constipation, nausea/vomiting; or if you are having problems with weight loss.

However, even the experts can't tell you exactly what is right for you. Each person's constitution is different, and you'll want to modify your diet according to what you can absorb and what makes you feel good.

Thankfully, your body provides you with an amazing feedback system. Listen to your body to figure out which foods satisfy your needs in which situations. For example, when you're thirsty your body sends you signals asking to be rehydrated. By listening and drinking healthy water, you are nurturing yourself.

This same type of mindfulness and intelligence can be brought to every aspect of your eating habits. With the first few bites of food, you may notice that certain foods on certain days just taste right. Temper your urge to indulge yourself and eat only what tastes "good" with an awareness of the benefits of a balanced diet or how you felt in the hours or days after eating certain foods or after eating too much.

Vitamins and Supplements

Should you take supplements? Generally, a balanced diet should cover all your needs except for vitamin D and calcium. If you're not getting daily direct sunlight on your skin, and especially if you live in a northern climate, then ingesting 1000–2000 IU of vitamin D every day is highly recommended.

In a study published in the *American Journal of Clinical Nutrition*, a group of healthy women in the northern United States who did not have cancer were followed for four years. The women assigned to taking 1100 IU of vitamin D daily reduced the risk of developing any cancer by 50 percent compared with those women taking a placebo. The women who took 1500 mg of calcium in addition to the vitamin D decreased their cancer risk even further.

To ingest the recommended daily calcium intake of 1500 mg usually means you will need to take calcium pills to supplement what is in your food.

3 • *Maintain a reasonable weight:* Your body is precious and the vehicle that allows you to extend your love into the world. Exercising, eating a healthy diet, and finding emotional balance should help you stay at a healthy weight. If you maintain too high a weight, try to decrease your daily caloric intake until you slowly start to lose the extra pounds. If you are underweight, try to increase your caloric intake each day.

Keeping your body's weight in balance can take a concerted effort and can be challenging but the health benefits are rewarding. If you need help, ask for direction from professionals. Support from loved ones can also be an important key to success in maintaining a healthy weight.

4 • *Sleep.* Sleeping at night in a darkened room allows your brain to produce hormones like melatonin that affect all the cells in your body.

Melatonin has been shown to suppress cancer cell activity in scientific experiments. Getting a good night's sleep will empower your body's innate ability to recover and provide you with more energy for your healing journey.

Talk to your doctor or even a sleep specialist for specific advice. Having a specific bedtime routine and other sleep-promoting habits, such as taking a warm bath before bed, listening to quiet music, reading a book, or practicing a relaxation technique will maximize your chance of a restful sleep.

5 • *Relaxation.* Practice a relaxation technique or a contemplative discipline every day. The key is to train your mind to settle down, allowing your body to relax as well. You can teach yourself any number of techniques which will elicit this relaxation response and facilitate awareness and psychological healing on your journey.

Many relaxation techniques have evolved out of the world spiritual traditions. For instance, meditation, prayer, and yoga not only connect you with the sacred aspects of life, but they also have profound health benefits.

As you read on you will learn a number of tools and skills you can continue to practice at home. You may also find it helpful to find an instructor, class or community which inspires you to practise relaxation every day.

Loving your Precious Body

Simple activities like taking a walk in nature or eating a meal slowly can also act as the gateway to appreciating the sacredness of life. For instance, if you are mindful while you are eating, you can be grateful for your food, experience the joy of eating, and really experience how special it is to be alive. As you begin to look at your body with this sense of gratitude, you'll naturally be drawn to take good care of it. Choosing to nurture yourself allows your wonderful body to walk out into the world, to extend a hand to others, and to give and receive a hug.

CHAPTER 9

Karen
Accepting and Aspiring

At the end of the Friday evening lecture and throughout the weekend Rob shares stories, like this one, about his experience as an oncologist and support group leader.

In *Love, Medicine and Miracles*, Dr. Bernie Siegel, the famous surgeon and support group advocate, describes the personality traits of his "exceptional cancer patients". Bernie noted that those people who did much better than expected were able to accept their diagnosis and find a deep sense of peace in their lives despite the outward challenges. Decades later, an increasing body of scientific literature supports Bernie's theory. Compiled medical reports of people undergoing spontaneous remissions of their cancers, and other "remarkable survivors", seem to support the power of acceptance.

But what does 'acceptance' really mean? Can we fully accept the distress that comes with a cancer diagnosis and still strive to heal?

Acceptance doesn't mean resignation. It is not an excuse to give up, or a passivity to let others make our decisions, or a wish that God would do everything for us. We still need to be proactive in our medical care and wise about how we spend our energy. Neither is acceptance meant to mask the emotional turmoil caused by a cancer diagnosis. Cancer can be the most trying experience of our lives.

Acceptance means looking directly at reality with mindful attention: "This is what is happening to me. This is how I feel." We gain greater clarity of the situation when we accept what is happening. With our feet firmly planted on the foundation of what is true right now, we can choose our next step more wisely. Conversely, not accepting or seeing the simple truth as our starting point is like walking in a fog so thick we can't see our feet.

My friend Karen is someone who tapped into the power of acceptance at a remarkably early phase of her breast cancer diagnosis. I was very close to Karen in medical school before she went on to become a nationally-respected anaesthetist, a wife, and a mother to two young children. We lost touch for a while, but over the last few years we began to exchange Christmas letters giving humorous updates on the lives of our young families.

A couple of years ago, when she had just turned forty, I received an email from Karen asking me to call her. I assumed that someone in her family had a cancer diagnosis, and she wanted some advice. As it turned out, Karen had found a lump in her breast and a suspicious mass in her armpit. Within days, a biopsy revealed locally advanced breast cancer. Fortunately it had not obviously spread to other parts of her body.

When I heard this news, tears welled up in my eyes. She had called me for advice about how to draw upon the body-mind-spirit connection as a complement to conventional care but, in those first moments when my voice began to break, it was Karen who consoled me just as she had many of her family and friends in the few short days since her diagnosis.

I was impressed with her matter-of-fact approach. When her friends would say to her, "I know you're going to beat this", she would respond with a gracious "Thank you" and then add that no one knows what is going to happen in the future. She knew exactly what was going on, was getting excellent care, and in her wisdom, she seemed comfortable with the uncertainty of what was to come.

Tired of explaining her philosophy to her many family members and friends, Karen sent out the following email to all her supporters:

"First of all, I want to thank you from the bottom of my heart for your expressions of concern and support. It means so much. Secondly, I want to reassure you that I am doing well—my spirits are good, my attitude positive. If you are interested in knowing more about where I am at, and where I have been, then read on. It may be a little bit raw, and a lot personal, so feel free to skip it if you're feeling squeamish.

…In finding a lump in my breast, then a mittful of lumps in my axilla during an idle moment sitting at my desk, I went from "life as I knew it" to the realization that I had an advanced stage breast cancer in less than 30 seconds. The next day, lying in the radiology suite for a series of core biopsies, with my three-year-old daughter in tow, I had the very real sense that this was happening to someone else. I saw two of the technicians exchange a look—that scrunched-mouth grimace of pity, a facial expression that says "What a sad case." I wanted to scream out "No, you don't understand. This is me. I'm a doctor. I'm a healthy person!"

But the ensuing week brought many discoveries, some painful, some wonderful. I have come to the belief that a large part of the shock of an experience like this comes from being forced to face one's mortality so clearly. Does any of us REALLY believe that we are going to die? Are we able to think about it and picture the seasons continuing to turn long after we are just dust? For some of us, I think, it is a hard place to go, and living our lives day to day demands that we tuck away that hard truth in order that we function in the quotidian.

But once I managed to accept that the reality of MY mortality had always been there, I could accept that nothing fundamental in my life had really changed with this diagnosis. I am still the same "me". My life has not changed drastically or dramatically. I am still here. I was not hit by a bus. My loved ones are still around me. Unbelievably, I can honestly say that I am as 'happy' now as I was five weeks ago. I am, even in this moment, missing a body part or two, hair about to fall out, completely and utterly whole. To be sure, I have different worries than before, and my time will be spent in ways that I had not anticipated. There is a large question mark about my health and my future. But again, I would argue that it was always there for me, as for all of us. It has now just struck me square in the face. Even the knowledge that the cancer had actually been there for five years or longer (EEK!) allows me to see the last few weeks, and the year ahead, as the first steps towards, rather than a plunge from, true wellness.

Few things in life are all good or all bad. One would think that winning twenty million dollars would bring unmitigated joy, but when one follows those "lucky" individuals five years down the road, it is clear that misery predominates. While I would erase my diagnosis in a minute if given the chance, I also recognize that it has brought me many gifts. My friends, family, and colleagues now express their love for me without hesitation. I feel a bit like Sally Field during her awful Oscar acceptance speech: "You like me! You really like me!" Regardless, it makes me feel surrounded with love in a way that I have never experienced before. All of the experiences of life have become more profound, more intense, more cherished. I have been able to give myself permission to focus exclusively on myself and my family, with nary a tinge of guilt.

Of course, it is not a bed of roses… While I really feel very little in the way of fear for myself, I am constantly thinking about my children. There is no positive spin to put on the scenario of two small children losing their mother. That part is so painful for me to contemplate that I cannot go there very often, nor for very long. But it does make me ensure that I give them the best of me that I can right now, that I love them with all the intensity that I feel. It also steels my resolve to fight this disease with everything I can. I will accept any treatment that shaves even a *fraction of a percentage point off my chance of recurrence, and God forbid, if recurrence comes, any treatment that will give me a single extra day. I am planning and working towards living until they have to send me to a nursing home at age 95 and I can make them feel guilty for not visiting me often enough.*

To this point, I have lived what I would describe as a 'charmed' life. No major hardships, many blessings. Sometimes we can lead ourselves to believe that we are totally in control of the path we are on, and that we are entitled to continue along that path as we wish. It is a rude awakening for someone like me to discover that I was connected to the general circumstances of my life by a gossamer-thin thread. When that thread snaps, with it comes the realization that ultimately, we control very little. What we can control are our actions, our attitudes, and our beliefs."

Karen is a wise woman who has worked with the process of accepting her situation and has come to make peace with it. At the same time, she is getting the best possible conventional medical care, and taking care of her body with healthy habits like exercise, a wholesome diet, and daily meditation.

But there is more to the story than simply accepting what is happening. She is in touch with the reality of the situation, and, at the same, she wants to be cured. Here is how Karen wrote about this aspiration:

"I suffered a couple of days of despair after the diagnosis. But since then I have known that I will be 'OK.' Maybe not 'OK' in the way that I would have defined it five weeks ago, but in a bigger sense. I felt that while I cannot be positive that I will 'beat this', I can be positive that I will have the courage to face what is ahead. I am positive that I will have the support from loved ones, the expertise from my doctors, and ultimately the grace from God to ensure that this turn in the road will not be a negative force in my life. And I believed all of that, and still believe that, from deep within my soul. But in the past two weeks, something else has crept in. I am starting to believe (or want to believe?) that I will 'beat this' in the conventional sense. I'm starting to demand it of myself, and to ask it of God. There is a proportion of women who survive breast cancer of my stage, so why not me?"

Accepting the reality of a cancer diagnosis while aspiring to be cured of it may sound conflicting — as if you are trying to go in two directions at once. Yet holding these two opposites at the same time is especially useful when working with the difficult emotions that arise with a cancer diagnosis and related treatments. It is normal to feel anger, sadness, frustration, guilt, pity, numbness, and a whole plethora of others emotions. These feelings can be particularly intense during the few weeks following a diagnosis. They often flare up again at the end of therapy, and can continue to well up for years. Instead of denying them or pushing them away, you can be open to these emotions and regard the whole process as an opportunity to heal on psychological and spiritual levels.

Karen accepts the uncertainty of her future, and is still determined to do everything she can to be there for her children. She continues to work with all her emotions as they arise each day, including truly loving herself as she is. By holding the tension of pro-activity and acceptance, both in her physical care and on the spiritual journey, she is nurturing her own transformation and healing.

Settling the Mind

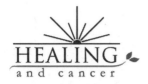

Saturday Morning • Settling the Mind

In this section of the book, you will listen to more inspiring stories, and learn essential healing skills rarely taught in the conventional medical system.

Recognizing your unique stress reaction and being able to settle your mind and body during the stressful phases of the cancer journey can make a tremendous difference in both your physical and psychological health. When your mind is settled, you are better able to appreciate all the goodness in the world that is both around you and within you.

Practicing mindfulness and meditation, as taught here, will help focus your attention on the practical issues of taking care of yourself, open you to the circle of giving and receiving, and, ultimately, deepen your awareness of the realm of spirit and the greater possibilities of healing.

At our website HealingandCancer.org you can watch full-length videos of the relaxation and visualization exercises, meditation, Qi Gong and Yoga taught at the retreat.

CHAPTER 10

The Power of Mindfulness

Life only unfolds in moments.
The healing power of mindfulness
lies in living each one as fully as we can.
Jon Kabat-Zinn

Saturday morning. *There is a positive buzz in the room as people find their way back to the healing circle. Some are excited to catch up with the people they met for the first time the previous evening. Others are still emotionally raw from listening to so many intimate stories all at once.*

They are all looking for something they can do that can really make a difference on the cancer journey, something powerful, simple and practical.

Drawing on his experience of observing his own mind during years of meditation practice, Tim starts the first lecture of the day by asking people to consider what they experience during a medical appointment:

What happened in your mind when you first heard "You have cancer" or when your doctor talked about treatment options, side effects and what might happen in the future?

When most people first confront the shock and uncertainty that come with a cancer diagnosis, a flood of thoughts goes through their minds like "Oh my God, what about my family? What am I going to do? What about work and our family finances? How is this going to affect my body? How am I going to tell everyone? I'm going to fight this with everything I've got. I can't believe this is happening to me!" and so on.

The first and most essential skill to learn in working with these racing thoughts and overwhelming emotions is 'Mindfulness'. The practice of mindfulness has been taught in the contemplative traditions of the East for thousands of years. By introducing mindfulness-based stress reduction, Dr. Jon Kabat-Zinn popularized the power of mindfulness practice in the west. As a young man, Jon was devoted to his daily meditation practice while working on a Ph.D. in microbiology. Seeing how helpful meditation was for his own wellbeing, he was inspired to offer mindfulness meditation and yoga to people who were suffering from chronic pain and other stress-related illnesses. The Mindfulness-based Stress Reduction Clinic began quietly in the basement of the University of Massachusetts Medical Center in 1979.

Patients were referred to Jon's eight-week program with various medical problems, often when their doctors had nothing else to offer them. Many of these people began to get better. Jon and his colleagues administered pre and post-clinic testing and published their impressive results in respected medical journals. Jon captured the essence of his teaching and the transformative stories of his patients in the best seller *"Full Catastrophe Living: Using the Wisdom of your Body and Mind to Face Stress, Pain and Illness."*

Health care professionals from around the world have attended teaching workshops lead by Jon and the stress reduction program has been replicated in hundreds of hospitals and clinics internationally. The medical literature now contains high-quality articles showing the benefits of mindfulness for every major medical illness, including cancer.

What is Mindfulness?

Mindfulness means deliberately paying attention. To be mindful is to be fully present in the here and now. Mindfulness is the discipline of training your mind to return to its natural alertness, unclouded by judgments, concepts and the confusion that can be caused by clinging to your thoughts. With mindfulness, you can be receptive, inquisitive and tuned into the richness of your senses to appreciate the richness of life.

Perhaps it's easier to explain mindfulness by showing its opposite. If you notice the nearly constant stream of thoughts going through your mind, you would probably find that much of the time your mind is not focussed on the present. You are either thinking about the past, such as rehashing a conversation from yesterday, or projecting into the future with vague hopes or worries. Your mind is somewhere else.

As an example, have you ever had that experience of driving to work, arriving at your desk, and thinking "How did I get here? I don't remember any of it: getting into the car, driving, parking, getting out and walking up the stairs." If this has happened to you, you were not present to the experience of driving because your mind was caught up in the waterfall of thoughts spilling through your head.

Separating Thoughts from Reality

Mindfulness also helps us see that our thoughts can separate us from the world around us. The philosopher Gregory Bateson said "The map is not the territory." To explain this idea, think of planning a romantic trip to France. Looking at a map and reading the travel guide about France would be vague and lifeless compared with the actual experience: walking through a cobblestoned town, hearing the village church bells ringing and dairy cows lowing, smelling lavender on the breeze, tasting the ripe grapes on the vine and the subtle flavours of wine and cheese, taking in the breathtaking views. Your actual trip is a feast of the senses; the map and guidebook are only someone else's one-dimensional views.

So think about your cancer map. The map here is your thoughts, opinions, and pre-conceived ideas of what is happening. If you focus on the map, you tend to experience a distorted version of reality made by your thoughts. Worrying excessively about cancer and what might happen in the future distorts your ability to be present on your journey. Learning that you don't always have to believe your thoughts is another important realization that comes with mindfulness practice.

Reconnecting our Minds to our Bodies

Not being mindful and living in our heads can also be harmful to our bodies. Often our minds and bodies are disconnected. The extreme version of disconnection in psychology is called *dissociation*. Mindfulness shows us that we all dissociate to some degree. When our minds are lost in thoughts and we are not present, we ignore the profound connection to our bodies.

Imagine a young couple with young children who have won a trip to Mexico for two. Their baby sitter quits on them at the last moment and they have no one to mind their children. They decide to go on the trip anyway, convincing themselves that "The kids will be alright. We'll only leave them for a week. We'll just get a lot of Cheerios and macaroni and cheese. They can watch TV and play video games. They'll be fine, right."

So they go to Mexico for a week and what happens? The house would be a total mess and maybe even burn down. The social workers would probably take the children into safe custody.

This is exactly what most of us do to our bodies. Our mind is on vacation, thousands of miles away, and no one is there minding the body. We need to pay attention to the needs of our bodies deliberately, from moment to moment.

Our bodies send us signals when we are thirsty and hungry, when we need exercise, and when we need sleep. We have a relationship with our bodies and, just as in all good relationships, we need to learn to listen. The more we train ourselves to listen, the more our bodies will tell us what to do. Sensitivity grows with time and effort so that we can pick up on more subtle messages guiding us towards health.

What do you do if the little red engine light on your car's dashboard starts to flash? Most of us take heed of this signal and take our car into a service station or we might look under the hood ourselves. We look deeply into it, to solve the root cause of the problem. By contrast what do we often do if we have a headache or back-pain? Most of us take a pill to make the symptoms go away. This approach is similar to putting a piece of duct-tape over the flashing light in your car so that it won't distract us while driving. Eventually it will lead to further problems and a breakdown of the system.

With mindfulness practice, we bring our attention back home into the body. Deliberate mindfulness works to repair important feedback loops that can heal patterns of disharmony in the physical systems that tend to go out of balance due to stress and illness. With mindfulness practice we can learn to love our bodies and love ourselves in this moment just as we are. When we do this we soften towards ourselves and natural healing begins to happen at all levels – uniting body, mind and spirit.

Mindfulness also Means Heart-fullness

In the east when people refer to mind, they often put their hand on the middle of their chest at the energetic heart center. When we bring mind-fulness into our lives, we are also cultivating loving kindness.

Although the practice of mindfulness has been shown, through rigorous science, to have a profound and positive effect on the brain, we are not just talking about what happens in our heads. From a bigger spiritual perspective, 'Mind' is really a boundless open system of intelligence that involves the body, the brain, the senses and the whole world perceived by the senses. Sometimes the word 'heart-fullness' is actually a better way to convey what we mean by mindfulness because it includes a quality of 'Heart': love, connection and gratitude for our world and our life.

Practicing heartfulness means deliberately cultivating your natural capacity to experience love and kindness as a powerful healing presence in your life. The emotional turmoil that comes with a cancer diagnosis often triggers old patterns of self judgement, fear and negativity. So many of us have a hard time truly accepting and loving ourselves in everyday life, let alone with the added stress of a major illness. With mindfulness we practice acceptance and non-judgement noticing our current state whatever that might be. We begin to notice the mental and emotional patterns that can cause further suffering. This mindful and heartful attention then arouses our natural intelligence and gradually we learn to let these patterns go. With time we also learn to accept and love ourselves just as we are in this very moment. This essential skill is like planting a seed of healing in your heart that grows daily as you nurture it.

Practical Benefits of Mindfulness

There are many practical benefits of practicing heartfulness and mindfulness on the cancer journey. As you practice, your ability to discern is sharpened and this helps you to negotiate the medical system, and choose a healthy lifestyle. Remembering to love yourself softens judgments, helping you to work with stressful situations, difficult thoughts, and disturbing emotions. Mindfulness gradually expands into awareness and arouses innate intelligence which guides the decisions you make, the words you speak, and the actions you take in life. Heartfulness helps you to feel connected in giving and receiving love.

Mindfulness may appear to be a very simple concept, yet to practice it can have a profound effect on every aspect of your life. If you think about it, the only time you actually have to live your life is right now. Only in this very moment can you experience joy, inspiration or compassion. Only in the present moment can you learn, love, heal and grow. With mindfulness, you heighten your awareness of the mystery of life as it unfolds.

CHAPTER 11

Bonnie
Learning to Paddle My Own Kayak

"How did I get myself into this?" Exhausted and scared, Bonnie fought through the waves and riptide to get back to shore.

The adventure that seemed to be the turning point in her recovery from cancer started innocently enough a couple hours earlier. On a warm July afternoon, on a beach in Maine, Bonnie kissed her husband on his cheek, waved to her friends and got into her own kayak. A petite woman with sparkling blue eyes, and curly greying hair, Bonnie sat up straight, and gripped her paddle with determination. She looked over at Karen, a friend and guide, and began paddling slowly, happy to spend some time alone reflecting on her life.

Her cancer journey had begun six years earlier at age 46, when her three kids were aged 16-23, and her career and passion as a corporate trainer was flourishing. She had noticed lumps in her neck and began to feel weak.

Her doctor called her with the results of a biopsy while Bonnie was running a seminar. "You have lymphoma and need to quit work today. Like… today!" Bonnie replied "I'm a trainer and I have many people here who have paid $10,000 a pop. I can't just walk out."

Her chemotherapy started three days later.

As Bonnie paddled along she recalled how hard it had been to tell her kids. Her eyes teared up as she thought about the long drive to visit her son at his boarding school to tell him the news in person. Her daughter was on exchange in Europe, and Bonnie couldn't hide her diagnosis from her any longer. They both cried and cried – Bonnie alone in her bedroom and her daughter in a phone booth in England.

Even while paddling, Bonnie realized that through six long years, on and off chemotherapy, the same worries were still ringing in her mind. "I just don't want to be a burden to anyone. My kids are in their mid-twenties. They should be out there leading their lives, not having to come home to a sick mother." Despite being in remission for over two years now, she still felt like her friends and family shouldn't have to deal with her diagnosis and that her kids should be out 'having fun'.

Bonnie set down her paddle and lowered her head. Karen interrupted her to ask if she wanted to go out farther, beyond the waves. Bonnie was quick to smile and agreed, despite feeling tired.

She had been tired for a long time and she couldn't figure out why. She has a loving husband and a large group of supportive friends. Hundreds of 'Get well' cards and letters line the walls and windows of the sunroom in her house. The sun shines through the cards pouring in the light of love and good wishes on her. But when she sees herself sitting in this room and thinks about how she has put on her 'Revlon face' to try to make everyone happy, she feels isolated and exhausted at her core.

As Bonnie turned to head to deeper water, the first wave caught her by surprise, splashing water in her face and stinging her eyes. She gritted her teeth and tried to dig in her paddle. As she struggled through the waves, she thought about the occasional turmoil she has had with her adult children. One day she said to her daughter, "Everyone in the family is just fed up with my lymphoma." Her daughter retorted in frustration "That's not true, Mom." Bonnie was still confused by the turbulence in their relationship and wondered how to make it better.

Bonnie was shocked out of her reflections by Karen who shouted "You're in a riptide." Bonnie looked up and noticed that her kayak was being pulled further and further away from her husband and friends on the shore. She realized she was going to have to get back over the waves and paddle against the tide to return to the beach. Karen shouted instructions: "I'm going to tell you what to do. But it's you who has to do it because you are in your own kayak."

Minutes passed as Bonnie circled in the riptide, frozen with indecision. Her skinny arms felt like lead. Her body began to shake in fear.

Finally, with a rush of adrenaline she shouted "Let's go" and paddled with all her might. "I paddled my little brains out. When I got to the shore, it was totally magical. My husband and our friends were on the shore and everyone was jumping around. I was yelling, 'I did it! I did it!'"

Months after her kayaking adventure, Bonnie reflected on the meaning of overcoming the waves and tide. "That was the turning point in my recovery from the cancer. It was a metaphor for how I needed to take care of myself. My paddling partner, she had to wait out there with me. Other people were waiting to see if I could do it. Then I realized I had to paddle my own kayak and not worry about everyone else."

Bonnie then went on to explain, despite this insight, she still struggles to justify caring for herself, giving an example of deciding to take an eight-week mindfulness course. "For my whole life I never felt I warranted the time for myself. I had work to do and kids, and I didn't feel I deserved anything just for me.

"With the lymphoma diagnosis, all of a sudden my time came. It became clear to me that learning mindfulness was exactly what I needed. They handed out audio tapes for practice and I set up a room for myself upstairs. It felt so good. And my family now knows when that door is shut I don't take phone calls, I don't receive visitors, I don't answer to 'what's for dinner?' When the door is shut, they know I'm doing my thing.

"And Yoga has been a lifesaver too. If I don't do yoga class a couple of times a week, I feel I'm losing not only my physical strength but also my mental strength. So when I get strung out or tired, when there's no reserve in the tank, I do some meditation and a couple of yoga poses and just pull myself together."

Bonnie then referred back to a question she had been asked earlier during the weekend retreat. "When Rob asked us what we really want to do, I had an epiphany. I thought about my life. Every day for the last 50 years, I have woken in the morning with the question 'What do I *have* to do today?'....not 'What do I *want* to do today?'

"Being a trainer for 30 years, every work day was focused on 'How can I make my client's day as good as possible'. My office was the training room. I never had a peaceful moment. I became a mom at 29 and from that moment on, I factored my family into every day's plan. And I am a wife, dog owner, daughter, sister, and friend too. I did not balance it very well, did I?

"I think I just figured out why I am so tired and why I need to take care of myself right now! Nobody else can paddle my kayak for me."

CHAPTER 12

The Raisin Eating Meditation

When experience is viewed in a certain way,
it presents nothing but doorways into the soul.
Jon Kabat-Zinn

Saturday morning. Silence falls over the room as fifty people slowly put a raisin to their lips.

Jon Kabat-Zinn devised the Raisin Eating Exercise in his stress reduction seminar to give people a sensory experience of being mindful rather than just talking about it. Each person in the group will eat a raisin slowly and mindfully as a way to show them that meditation is not something that is mystical or otherworldly. On the contrary, mindfulness meditation is about being grounded and fully present in the here and now—in the midst of our complex lives.

As the raisins are passed out, Tim gives instructions: "Take one small raisin and begin by experiencing it fully with all of your senses. Feel it with your fingers, look at its peculiar wrinkly shape with your eyes, smell the faint scent, place it on your lips and really feel it, and finally taste it. But don't start chewing right away. Take the time to just feel it in your mouth, moving it around with your tongue and noticing the textures and everything else."

Each person will experience eating a single raisin in a different way. Sue, who has a diagnosis of multiple myeloma, and who has already outlived her doctor's predictions by years, looks like a little girl brimming with delight as she rubs the raisin against her lips. Kathy, a former executive who faces a dual diagnosis of liver disease and Hodgkin's lymphoma, has a peaceful, almost sacred look on her face as she closes her eyes and slowly moves the raisin around in her mouth.

Everyone is being drawn deeply into the sensations generated by millions of nerve endings in the lips, nose, and mouth. In the one-pointed attention of eating a raisin mindfully, faces soften as the cares of the world fall away. An energy of simple joy pervades the room.

After a few minutes Tim rings little Tibetan cymbals to mark the end of this short meditation. Looking to the group he asks "So, what did you notice?"

People slowly shift from a contemplative inner feeling to the very different activity of putting that experience into thoughts and words. The deep silence fades as the noise in everyone's mind starts up again.

The first one to speak is Julian, a tall man sitting at the back of the room. He has incurable prostate cancer and has continued to practice meditation throughout his journey. He holds his arms out as wide as he can and says, "My raisin was THIS BIG." The group laughs in appreciation.

Tim responds, "That's great. The bigness of your raisin attests to the bigness of your mindfulness. The attention that you put into it is really what makes the difference."

Diane, a bright-eyed woman undergoing chemotherapy for ovarian cancer, chimes in, "There is such a difference in texture between the outside and the inside of a raisin. At first, when I rolled it around, it was very rough, hard, and dry, but I could feel that there was fruit on the inside. Then, when I slowly bit into it, the inside was very fruity, moist, and soft. I could taste the grape that is now inside the raisin. That's something I hadn't noticed before."

"Aha!" Tim smiles. "Isn't that interesting? So much experience in just one little raisin."

Cory chimes in with the next observation. A 75-year-old woman with soft rosy cheeks, warm eyes and a lilting Dutch accent, she spent seven years nursing her husband through multiple myeloma before being diagnosed with breast cancer herself. A broad smile appears on her face. "I love raisins. I never really realized how rough a raisin is - when you wrap your tongue around it, and really feel all those little ridges, it's really rough. Usually I just take a handful and, bingo, they're gone!"

"So you experienced the roughness and the wrinkles?" Tim asks. "Yes," she continues. "Those wrinkles on the raisin, they reminded me of my face!" The whole group bursts out laughing.

"You're gorgeous!" Tim adds. "You have a beautiful face."

Next, a woman with short red hair and dark glasses sheepishly admits, with a wide grin, "I don't think I stayed in the present, because the raisin kept reminding me of the raisin cake my mother used to make. And rice pudding with raisins. I just kept thinking of food." There is more laughter as many participants acknowledge having a similar experience.

Tim points out, "So that's something interesting to notice also. We can be mindful of our mind as it pulls us into memories and away from sensing the raisin in the present. You can be mindful of your memories, taking you out of the present for an instant, but if you can pay attention to that as it happens, then your mindfulness is still present. You can observe the memories. You may know of the book 'The Remembrance of Things Past', by Marcel Proust, where just one little memory takes him off for 200 pages of flashbacks, and then finally he comes back to the initial moment."

The next person to speak is a woman with breast cancer, sitting behind a walker, who shared her religious beliefs with the group during opening circle the day before. "I was just wondering if anyone remembered to say grace before they ate their raisin?"

Tim responds to her question about grace. "I like to say that mindfulness is the opposite of taking things for granted. We go through most of our lives in a trance-like state, half asleep. We look at our watch, impatiently counting the hours and thinking, 'Ho hum. Another day.' We don't realize what a miracle it is simply to be alive, breathing fresh air and getting enough to eat each day. So many conditions have to come together in just the right way to make this moment of life possible.

"When we are mindful, we align ourselves with the natural sacredness of things just as they are. We can eventually recognize that existence itself is a state of grace, and gratitude becomes our path toward natural appreciation and joy."

Then a cheerful woman with an English accent excitedly adds, "I think I can see great diet success with this mindfulness approach. I felt almost the same intensity with one raisin as eating my favourite Christmas pudding. I love Christmas pudding, and I could have eaten a whole bowl full of it in the same time that it took me to get the same pleasure out of that one raisin. Now that is a diet success."

"Great point," Tim responds. "I think mindfulness is probably one of the most important things for nutrition and dieting and for taking good care of your body. Your body knows what's good for you and how much is good for you. Isn't it wonderful that, with more attention, you can get as much pleasure out of one raisin that you might get from a dish that has hundreds more calories? With mindfulness, one raisin becomes a great dessert."

Cynthia nods in agreement. Neatly dressed, with close-cropped curly blond hair, she had been diagnosed with ovarian cancer just over a year ago. Earlier in the weekend she had expressed to the group how afraid she has been, and how much she has felt that cancer "shakes up your whole world". She speaks slowly in a soft and melodious voice. "I think often, with food, I have cravings, and when I try to satisfy that craving, I eat. But then when the food is gone, I'm still dissatisfied because I want more. I think a lot of that has to do with not paying attention to what you are doing when you are actually eating in the first place, so, when it's finished you are still craving."

Tim continues. "Never really being satisfied is a common theme in our society. As soon as something is finished, we want another experience to satisfy our constant craving. Craving itself has become a habit, irrespective of what we are craving. Even when we get what we want, we start to think that maybe that is not quite what we wanted and again we are dissatisfied. We end up constantly grasping at the outside world, looking for it to fulfill a yearning within us that, perhaps, it cannot fulfill.

"Where does real contentment come from? Perhaps, if we receive reality as it unfolds, with mindfulness, we might find that it is already enough – it fulfills us. We yearn for this simple contentment: to be at peace, to be satisfied, to feel good with things just as they are. Yet contentment is an attitude that we can cultivate from the inside. This key ingredient to fulfillment is so simple it is easy to overlook."

Joyce speaks next. A small woman with stage three colon cancer, she looks as if she has the inner strength of a pioneer. "I think part of the pleasure, for me, was that we were all doing the same thing at the same time. I think so much of our experience is different for all of us at any given moment. Whereas just now, eating that raisin in silence together, just for that short time, there was community. Even though we were probably all thinking different things while chewing, still we were in communion with one another."

"That's a wonderful observation," Tim responds. "I actually had that same thought: that when you synchronize everybody together, doing the same thing at the same time, a kind of oneness of mind happens. Similarly, that is why group meditation practice is powerful. A feeling of true community is something we all need more in our lives. It is healing to feel part of something that is alive and vibrant, growing and evolving—something bigger than ourselves."

Nancy speaks next. She is struggling in her recovery from a rare gynecological cancer. She has recently been laid off from her job and admits to struggling in her relationships. She is alone and very much wants a life partner and a fulfilling career, but all this has been put on the back burner with her treatment. Now, with cancer, her whole world seems to be caving in on her, yet she bravely goes forward. "Savouring that raisin, for me, was a reminder to savour life."

The group is perking up. Tim continues "It is so true; every moment of our life is just like that little raisin. Each moment has so much to offer. Every moment of our life is full of potential richness, insight, and wisdom – if we're really paying attention.

"It's like a good novel. Good writers are mindful of the details. They live their lives the same as we do, but they are noticing things carefully and they don't take the little things for granted. They pick up on the quirky connections between what might otherwise seem meaningless. In their writing, they extract from those little details all this fascinating meaning – meaning that seems hidden to most of us. Whether the story or the novel is dark and painful or pleasant and celebratory, tragic or comic, it doesn't really matter. We still read it or we watch the movie because the writer has been mindful of the details and has thereby drawn out the truth and fullness of life. We can do that too. We can live our lives with that same kind of artfulness and deep meaning."

The next morning, during 'check-in' period, Kathy, the semi-retired executive, started the group discussion, "What I kept going over last night was the raisin exercise. I thought about eating that raisin. And you'd think it was just a raisin, for heaven's sakes! But it was much more. It was Christmas pudding, a lesson in gratitude, a flashback in a novel, and a long, long moment of ecstasy. During supper last night, not only was I enjoying the food more, but every moment seemed like it could expand for me. Every moment, every relationship, every conversation can be like that. Dying is not my biggest fear—it's *not having lived*. That's huge for me."

Cynthia added to Kathy's insights. "Sometimes something as small as a raisin can shift your whole view of life and remind us that our experiences are always two-sided. On the one side, there is the pain of dealing with cancer physically and mentally. There is the doubt, the fear, and all the things that go along with the diagnosis.

"On the other side, cancer has been a huge gift. Sometimes that gift is being in a state of grace - grace to be mindful of the love that people bestow on us, and mindful of our friendships.

"We can learn to have the gratitude for the world that we live in, the beauty that surrounds us in every single day—to fully experience that, like we did with that little raisin. Just imagine being mindful of the gift that is this life, this world and especially the people we share our lives with from day to day. A little dried-up raisin can be a beautiful thing."

CHAPTER 13

Coming Home to Your Body
Mindful Breath and Body Scan

Change .... starts with being willing to have a
compassionate relationship with the parts of ourselves that
we feel are not worthy of existing on the planet. If we
are willing through meditation to be mindful not only
of what feels comfortable, but also of what pain feels like,
if we even aspire to stay awake and open to what we're
feeling, to recognize and acknowledge it as best we can in
each moment, then something begins to change.
Pema Chrödrön

*Saturday morning. People of all shapes and sizes are lying on yoga mats on
their backs with their knees up in the air and their feet flat on the floor. Lying
down higgledy-piggledy all over the room or sitting in chairs, they are interwoven
with a colourful array of blankets, pillows, and carrying bags. It looks like nap
time at a pre-school except for the fact that most everybody here is over forty.*

*They have just finished the raisin eating meditation and are now tuning into the
breath with the same deliberate mindfulness they experienced in tasting the raisin.
Everyone has a hand on their chest and a hand on their belly and Tim asks them
to sense exactly how they breathe.*

Though most of us know we are over-stressed, we are not usually aware
of the level of stress and bodily tension we carry day-by-day. In the same
way that a fish doesn't realize it's swimming in water, our chronic stress is
unquestioned and all pervasive. But when we practice deep states of relaxation we start to notice the stark contrast between being more fully relaxed
and our habitual state of rigid tension and hyper-arousal that we take as the
norm. Without deliberate practice, we may never experience what deep relaxation feels like. Practicing mindful breathing and the mindful body scan
meditation are key to reducing stress and promoting healing on all levels.

Mindful Breathing

We start with mindfulness of the breath. Take a moment right now and ask yourself: How am I breathing? Scan your body to find the actual sensations of breathing – not your *thoughts* about the breath but the actual *sensations* of the air going in and out, along with your bodily movements of breathing. Try not to change your breathing in any way to make it more perceptible or to breathe in some way you think is correct. Simply, let the breath be as it is, and observe it with great care and curiosity.

If you notice your chest expands and contracts with each breath, then you are probably somewhat caught up in a pattern of chronic stress. Chest breathing is necessary and helpful during aerobic exercise or if you suddenly need to muster up your energy, but, if you are at rest, then shallow chest breathing is not very efficient and it can feed the physiology of chronic stress.

Unfortunately, most people in our highly stressed society are shallow chest breathers and rarely use their diaphragm as the primary means of breathing. The diaphragm is a dome-shaped muscle that acts as a partition between your chest and abdominal contents. In healthy diaphragmatic breathing, the expansion and contraction of the diaphragm acts like a bellows to fill and expel air from the lungs.

If you find that you are a shallow chest breather, don't be hard on yourself. You are not alone. Becoming aware of your shallow chest breathing is the first step in transforming your breath. Learning diaphragmatic breathing is a powerful way to re-set your autonomic nervous system by stimulating a particular bundle of nerves in the belly. This, in turn, begins the relaxation response that affects your whole body.

Try to sense what is happening inside at the base of your ribs, belly and pelvic region as you breathe. With healthy belly breathing, as you take a breath in, the surface of your diaphragm presses downward. Relaxing the abdominal muscles a bit allows the belly to expand as you inhale. As you exhale, both the diaphragm and abdominal muscles will return to the resting position.

As you start to retrain your system into this more healthy way of breathing, it is helpful to exaggerate it and to be extra mindful. For example, on the in-breath, you may imagine or feel like you are blowing up a balloon in your belly or as if you have a pregnant belly. As you breathe in more deeply, you may even get the sense of pushing the air deep into your pelvis as if you are pushing a baby out. On the out-breath, just relax, let go completely, and your belly will fall again. Your chest should remain quiet throughout the breathing cycle.

Once you start to get the feeling for belly breathing, it is helpful to add 'a pelvic tilt' to the breathing movements in your body. This way your lower spine and pelvis are involved in breathing. It is easiest to do a pelvic tilt on a mat on the floor with your knees up in the air and your feet flat on the floor.

You can also do a pelvic tilt while breathing and sitting in a chair. Start by placing yourself in a comfortable and upright position. Move your bottom forward a couple of inches on the chair. Your back should not be touching the back of the chair. Lean your chest toward your thighs a little bit, and then, as you sit back upright again, arch your lower back slightly. Lift up the center of your chest a little and straighten the back of your neck so the very top of your head is drawn towards the sky. You may notice that this is the same basic posture you use for sitting meditation in a chair. Be mindful of the natural S-curve of your spine, especially the curve in the lower back.

Now that you're in position, you can begin the pelvic tilts while doing your belly breathing. You can also think of the pelvic tilt as arching and flattening your lower spine with each breathing cycle. As you breathe in, you actually start to arch your lower back a little bit more than usual while your belly expands.

The other way to think about it is to stick your bum out slightly on the in-breath. Then as you breathe out the curve in your lower back will straighten a bit and your belly will fall. Sitting upright in a chair you may notice that you get a little taller on the in-breath and a little shorter on the out-breath as your spine begins to move and flex with the flow of the breath. As you get the hang of this you might notice a gentle wave motion in your spine.

When we pay attention to breathing, we can see that there are actually four stages to the breath: the in-breath; a slight pause of fullness and transition;, the out-breath;, and a slight pause of emptiness and letting go. See if you can be mindful of this natural rhythm in the breath as you feel a slight wave-like motion in your lower spine.

You do not have to force these movements. Let the breath initiate and guide these gentle motions in your spine and belly. This is the way a baby breathes naturally from birth. Once you engage this way of breathing again, your body will take over and come back home to what it knows as a calm and relaxed state. Be patient with yourself if you have been a shallow chest breather or have not used your diaphragm to breathe for decades; it may take mindful effort to turn those habit patterns around.

Body Scan

It is easiest to do a body scan while lying on a mat on the floor with your legs out straight, arms at a comfortable distance from your sides with palms facing up. This is a yoga posture, known as savasana, and is a pose of deep relaxation and peaceful breathing that allows the cells in one's body to heal. Even without doing yoga first, this simple posture is very beneficial. By being present to the sensations and feelings in your body, you can begin to reconnect the feedback loops that the body depends on to foster optimal health.

You can modify this lying position with pillows under your knees and head for comfort, or even do the scan while sitting in a chair or recliner.

The body scan is like sitting meditation in that it trains your mind to bring your attention back, over and over, into the present moment and to the sensations in your body. By tuning into each part of the body with mindfulness, you are bringing the healing power of your attention into each area. You can begin to truly make friends with your body.

As an analogy, if you ignore or mistreat your friends they will tend to drift away or even become difficult or hostile. Your body is no different.

Cultivating a healthy relationship with your body is like cultivating any other healthy relationship. You start with a clear and deliberate intention and then use the power of your mindful attention to stay connected and to listen carefully to the needs of your friend - your own body.

At the retreat, a participant shared a well-known French expression which describes perfectly the purpose and practice of the body scan. She said that the body scan helped her to feel: "*Bien dans sa peau*," or "Good in your skin." She explained further that this phrase means to be fully comfortable with yourself, so that you radiate a sense of ease, peace and contentment. She also said that when you feel good in your own skin on a very deep level, then others will feel that as well. When they are around you they feel good too. *Bien dans sa peau* means being relaxed, fully present, balanced and natural. It means there is a good connection between your body and your soul.

The body scan begins by feeling those places of contact where the body touches the floor or the mat, mindfully tuning into the actual sensations of pressure in your heels, calves, thighs, buttocks, back, shoulders, neck and head. Being mindful of the physical sensations created by lying on the floor can help tame your wild mind and allow you to anchor it directly in the concrete experience of your physical sensations. Reestablishing your simple, direct and natural connection to the earth can be profoundly healing.

Normally throughout our busy lives, we are caught up in our own agendas. We speed about resisting gravity, pulling and pushing ourselves in opposition to its power in our life. We may even think of gravity as a force that slows us down. However, the body scan teaches us that with deep relaxation and mindfulness we can gradually learn to be grounded. This means that you can begin to experience gravity and the physical presence of the earth as a very positive power in your life.

During the body scan, you can release stress, emotional confusion and your busy mind, letting it all go, as if drawn by gravity to be absorbed into the earth. This teaches you to let go of your habitual resistance of pulling away from gravity and start to give in to the feeling of comfort that comes from being held by mother earth.

Practicing Relaxation and Being Present

Relaxation is something that requires practice. If you have spent most of your life training yourself to be stressed, it takes deliberate undoing to train your body to find progressive states of deep relaxation. When you practice the body scan, don't be alarmed if you find that all you feel is that you can't relax and that your mind is running all over the place. It takes a consistent effort to turn this all around.

In meditation training, we often use the phrase "monkey mind" to describe the wild mind. It is like a monkey swinging all over the place, going off in random directions for pure entertainment, and hardly ever being still. When we train ourselves in patience and perseverance through mindfulness practice, gradually we begin to tame the monkey mind and gradually there is more synchronization between body and mind. The main point is to always try to come back to the immediate concrete presence of your physical form on the mat or in the chair, if only for an instant.

Even when you think it is not working or when you think that you are not doing it right, let go of those judgments just as you let go of the monkey mind.

The simple acts of mindful breathing, scanning the body and practicing relaxation on the yoga mat can reduce stress and tap into the body's reservoir of intelligence and wisdom. When internal knots of tension become untangled, then one's natural energy can flow more freely and promote healing.

CHAPTER 14

Cathy
Learning to Listen to Myself

A sense of peace envelops Cathy as she sits back to listen to the five other women in her small group. The question arises whether the cancer diagnosis can be a gift, and Cathy leans forward to join the discussion. A 36-year-old mother of two teens, her dark brown hair has grown in curly after chemotherapy for lymphoma, and her blue eyes are penetrating yet calm.

A blur of images rushes across her mind before she shares her story with the group. She's back as a little girl, age nine, standing over her five year old sister who has been crying – Cathy is stroking her hair late at night. Their parents have divorced and their mom has moved away. She is telling her little sister, "It's going to be fine. I'll take care of you." These words echo over and over as her life flashes by.

A second image from a year ago comes up. Her girls, ages 14 and 12, are frantically cleaning up the house before a family get-together. Her mom and step-father are pulling up in the driveway. The house is immaculate. Nothing is out of place - nothing that they can use to judge her. Cathy runs up the stairs to dry the drips of water in the sink. She opens the front door, panting through a smile.

As the images fade, her thoughts emerge and her story begins. "I think cancer has been a gift for me because my life before cancer was really stressful. I worked for my sister and step-dad in an insurance brokerage. I was hired as the receptionist to open the mail and answer the phones. But I ended up doing things like bank deposits and payables. With my phobia of math, I was always tense because I didn't want to cost the company by making a mistake. I was the 'go to' girl. If you had something that you needed done, you could ask me.

"Every day it was 'go, go, go'. I got up at 5:30 to go to the gym because I weighed 222 pounds and would have given my arm to be thin. From the gym, I went to work with phones ringing all day, standing in line ups at the bank. Then it was always 'go, go, go'. I was stressed. I had to be home at 3 o'clock when my youngest came home from school. She has a developmental coordination disorder and can't take care of herself. Get home. OK homework, OK dinner, OK whatever's happening tonight. OK bedtime at 9 o'clock. It was crazy.

"A year ago I was starting to have diarrhea and this pain in my gut." Another image appears from the past. At a school council meeting, Cathy hunches towards the table, exhausted, placing her hand over her aching stomach. The Chair of the meeting is asking for someone to be Vice-Chair and looks to Cathy to volunteer. Cathy straightens up and a familiar sense of guilt floods over her. She has always said 'yes.' In her mind she knows she can't do it but instead the words "I'll do it" spill out. Everyone smiles.

Cathy looks to the discussion group and continues her story. "The pain in my gut got worse. I could hardly eat anything and was losing weight. Everyone thought I looked great. But I'd go into my sister's office in tears. She kept telling me to see my doctor. So finally I did. I had a cat scan that showed a 12 by 7cm mass wrapped around the blood vessels in the middle of my gut."

Cathy remembers the scene in the surgeon's office. Her husband, mom and sister are looking nervous and Cathy tries to joke with them. The surgeon tells them he'll arrange for a biopsy and starts to leave but Cathy insists he tell her what he thinks the mass is. "Well, we think it's a lymphoma." The blood drains from her face. Her first thought is "I have cancer. Oh my God."

Cathy wants to burst into tears but she can see her mother and sister are already crying. Her grandmother died of lymphoma in her early fifties when Cathy was seven years old. Looking to her husband, whose eyes are wide in disbelief, Cathy squeezes her fists to suppress the trembling in her shaking hands. She squints and clenches her jaw for her family to see.

"I was sick but I felt I had to pretend it wasn't happening. But I kept asking myself 'What's going to happen with my kids, and my husband? What does this all mean?' It was just surreal.

"The biopsy did prove it was a type of lymphoma called diffuse large B cell." She pauses as she sees the mental picture of first meeting her oncologist. It's evening, lying in the hospital bed on morphine, she is chatting with her mom and sister. A young Chinese man, dressed in a green disposable smock, walks in and tells them she has an aggressive form of cancer and will soon start on chemotherapy. Compelled to be loving, even in the most difficult circumstance, she gets off the bed and gives this small doctor a hug.

"I started a new chemotherapy protocol called CHOP-R. I got chemo every two weeks rather than the usual way of every three weeks. Chemo was hitting me hard and I was vomiting, dizzy, and exhausted. I couldn't handle any type of noise, including my kids laughing and playing. My husband started working from home to be with me."

Up flashes the image of her hair falling out and the decision to shave her head. Her mom and youngest daughter help her. Her eldest daughter wants nothing to do with it. Afterwards, when Cathy is alone, she looks in the bathroom mirror. Terrified, she starts sobbing.

"The chemo wasn't shrinking the tumor so they gave me more. I got every complication in the book. Everything, even lemonade, made me throw up. The doctors talked about putting me on an IV to feed me. At times, I was so low that I thought that there was nothing else God could throw in my face.

"I was wrong." Cathy relives the first few hours of the scariest day of her life. At home, on a Saturday morning, Cathy awakes to the sound of her girls chatting downstairs. Pulling on the handrail of her bed to sit up, Cathy feels dizzy, as if she's hung over. Struggling with the tie on her yoga pants, she walks downstairs to pour a glass of pink lemonade. But she can't stand up. She slumps onto the sofa.

Her sister Kerry arrives to take her for a drive and looks shocked 'Are you OK?' Cathy wants to say "I'm fine, damn it. Now can you please help me with my yoga pants," but all that comes out is "Mish, Mish."

Kerry gets Cathy's husband to try to stand her up but Cathy falls back like a dead weight. Cathy keeps shouting at them in her mind "There's nothing wrong with me" but they don't understand. Her girls are looking scared. Cathy is trapped inside. She can't fix this problem - can't make everything OK again. Lying there as a lump on the stretcher, the paramedics carry her away. She looks up at her girls — horrified by the fear in their faces.

Cathy explains "I had a stroke. I couldn't move. The only thing I could say was 'Thank you.' I thought everyone was taking it much too seriously. I didn't want to be a bother.

"I was hooked up to machines. My blood pressure started to drop and I was sent to the ICU. The nurses didn't think I was going to make it. The doctor took my husband and sister aside and asked if I should be resuscitated if my heart stopped. My sister shouted at him 'She's only 36 years old.'"

"I desperately wanted to live. I would wake up in the morning and force myself to make it until evening. I kept thinking 'what would my family do without me?'

"After four days in ICU, I was transferred back to the cancer floor. I was so weak I couldn't even turn my head. I had a catheter in my bladder and a feeding tube down my throat; I was wearing a diaper and still throwing up a dozen times per day. Worst of all I couldn't communicate." Cathy shudders as she relives the nightmare of her time on the ward: "I had intense cramps in my pelvis. I was writhing in pain and crying uncontrollably but I couldn't explain what was happening. My sister ran to the nurses to get help. Two days later, the palliative care doctor figured out I was having bladder spasms.

"I couldn't speak so nobody would listen to me and I wanted to give up. In the darkness of the hospital room, I had a breakthrough realization: I felt that nobody had listened to me for most of my life. Things had to change and I had to learn to speak up.

"The surgeons operated to remove a kink in my bowel. Luckily there was no cancer, and I began to eat again. But I was so weak my sister had to shave my legs, and cut and paint my nails. These were things that I would have never expected anybody to do for me. I felt I was an inconvenience. Fortunately, the only thing I could say was 'Thank you' and I said it a lot."

The group is entranced with this story, wondering how, only a few short months since this horrible ordeal, Cathy could look so radiant. "I started getting stronger. My hair and eyebrows started coming in. My mom brought in my make-up and clothes from home. I pushed myself to walk around the ward using my walker – three laps, three times per day. My speech was coming back. The nurses called me the miracle girl. I knew every one of them, knew about their kids, and their hobbies - we really cared about each other.

"After 13 weeks in hospital, I got to go home with my walker and a commode. Yahoo! My girls and husband were happy but I was mortified that my husband had to clean out my commode.

"But I started giving in to receiving help. My perfectionist ways were melting away. One day I spilled a cup of tea beside the couch and instead of thinking 'Oh, that was stupid' I calmly said to myself 'Honey, it's not going to work to put tea on the floor.' It was the kind mothering voice I used with my kids- but a voice I had never before used on myself.

"Two weeks after I left the hospital, I was readmitted. I was dehydrated from diarrhea and had a fever. I had a super bug called C. Difficile and was started on antibiotics. They did more scans. I started to get nervous because they weren't telling me what the scans were showing. One afternoon the palliative care doctor came in looking gloomy. I thought 'This is not good.'

"She told me the cancer had spread to my bowel. I thought 'OK, I'll just fight harder'. But the doctor said they couldn't treat the cancer because I was too weak to have chemotherapy. She told me if I was strong enough to walk, I could get a feeding tube and stay at home until I became bed-ridden - when I would come back in to the hospital to die. It was the first time I really thought about dying and the first time I admitted that there was something I couldn't fix."

Cathy vividly remembers thanking the palliative care doctor and waiting until she left before breaking down. "Minutes after the doctor left, my sister walked in. Through sobs, I told her 'I can't see you. Leave. Get out! Get out! Go get the doctor.' My sister found the doctor and learned the bad news for herself. When she returned twenty minutes later, she lay on the bed beside me and said, 'We have been together since I was born. We're not losing you now.'

"That moment helped me realize that this is about me. That was my gift. Someone up there, or whatever you want to call it, put me in these spots so I could finally learn to listen and care for myself - and not worry about everybody else. Everybody else is important, everybody else is special, everybody else needs me to some degree, but I need me too."

Cathy pauses. "It was amazing yesterday, when we were on the yoga mats and doing the body scan, and Tim said 'Listen to your body,' I had this overwhelming thought that "yes, I'm a cancer survivor and, yes, I'm a cancer sufferer, but I realized I'm also a cancer listener." I've learned so much by listening to my body and listening to how I really feel – it has been an awakening."

Someone in the group remembers that during the opening circle Cathy had said that now there are no signs of cancer, and asks "What happened?"

Cathy continues. "A special scan was ordered and it showed the tumor was actually shrinking and the bowel swelling seen on the CAT scan was caused by inflammation. It was benign. I was thrilled!

"But the shock of having been told I was 'terminal' had changed something in me. Even after the good news, I kept thinking about the purpose of life and if my family could cope without me."

Cathy's thoughts flash back to a time in hospital when her mother dropped in unexpectedly one evening. Cathy had started to plan her funeral in her head and, in a rare moment of vulnerability, asks her mother: 'Have I made a difference in others' lives? Will I be remembered? Will my girls really know who I am or will they forget about me? Who will come to my funeral? Will they come out of obligation or because I touched them in some way?' Cathy's mom holds her hand and they cry and laugh together.

"Then early one morning, just as the sun was rising up over the horizon and shining on my wall, I had this strange feeling of not being alone, even though I was the only person in my room. The IV machine was making its ticking sound and I felt oddly relaxed and at peace with life. I had this inexplicable feeling of being held in a big embrace. It was like I was a little girl again and my daddy was swinging me up and encompassing me in a giant bear hug.

"That was the first time in my life I had felt safe and secure and not alone. I instantly recognized this was a hug from God, and He has been with me the entire time. I just needed faith that He was with me. At that moment my life changed. So now, even when I am by myself or feeling lonely, I know I am not alone. That moment gave me the permission to be my own self and now I can say 'I need help.'" A feeling of gratitude overcomes Cathy as she reflects on all the help she received from her family, her friends and all the doctors and nurses during her long recovery.

Cathy remembers that sometimes help comes in unusual ways. After getting an infection called C. Difficile, Cathy suffered from months of diarrhea, despite several courses of antibiotics. Losing weight and becoming weaker and weaker, fortunately, she was referred to a world expert in infectious diseases. This medical expert explained that her diarrhea was caused by a lack of normal bacteria in her intestines to fight off the superbug.

This doctor instructed her to insert a sample of stool from her mother and sister into her own rectum, in a process called a fecal transplant. Cathy recalls the necessary preparations for this and, in particular, a disgusting brown mixture she had poured into an enema bottle on her bathroom counter. While the memory makes her cringe, the procedure proved to be successful and she is grateful both to the science of medicine and to her mother and sister for helping her.

Cathy smiles as she updates the group, "The doctors tell me my scans are clear but I have a fifty percent chance of recurrence. All I know is my health is slowly improving. I'm holding steady at 148 lbs. I'm injecting myself with a blood thinner twice daily to prevent another stroke, and taking a special pain pill for the pins and needles in my hands and feet I got from the chemotherapy. I see an acupuncturist every two weeks, and a naturopath once a month. I am eating properly and exercising too, taking vitamins and listening to my body.

"And I'm much more relaxed." Cathy smiles to herself as she remembers a scene from the previous week. Her girlfriend is on the phone, inviting her to come over for coffee. Cathy looks into the bathroom where she can see towels strewn on the floor and splatters on the mirror. Turning her back, she grabs a sweater and says 'I'll be right over. The housework can wait.'

"I've also learned to say thank you to everything. If it is a clogged sink, instead of freaking out I just look up to the sky and say 'Thank you. Thank you so much for letting me be here. Thank you for all of the lessons I'm learning. And thank you for loving me.' That's all that's important in the whole scheme of things – loving and feeling loved – truly loved.

"I feel like I have one foot in the physical world and one foot in the spiritual world. I am doing courses in The Healing Journey and thinking about things I would never have thought about before, like how important I am to those who love me. And that I am good enough – although I still struggle with that. I think about dying and living, and God, and the ways of the universe, and friends, and the impact I have on everything in my life. It goes on and on.

"Giving myself permission to think like this, I can see more clearly what is going on around me. Like last week, when I was out walking, I saw a bud blooming on a lilac tree. I stopped and smelled it. It was so exciting.

"I have also realized things do not have to be perfectly in order. The imperfections are already perfect and the way they should be. I feel like my blinders have been taken off and finally I can see."

CHAPTER 15

Why Meditate?

Experiences of wholeness are as accessible to people with chronic illness or stress-related problems as they are to anyone else. Moments of experiencing wholeness, moments when you connect with the domain of your own being, often include a palpable sense of being larger than your illness or your problems and in a much better position to come to terms with them.
Jon Kabat-Zinn

Saturday morning. As *Tim guides the group in one of several brief meditation sessions throughout the weekend, the room is enveloped in a calm and vibrant energy. Afterwards Tim gives a talk about the value of meditation.*

Physiological Benefits of Meditation

The benefits of meditation include improvements in all aspects of physical health – heart, gastrointestinal, hormonal, and especially the immune system. Studies with people affected by a cancer diagnosis show that practicing mediation improves their mood, decreases anxiety, anger and confusion – and gives them more vigour for life. They feel less stressed, have more energy, are less likely to suffer debilitating emotional ups and downs, and feel they can concentrate better.

The experience of calm while meditating has a physiological basis: the electrical circuitry in your brain actually changes. The activity in some areas of the brain slows down while other areas, like the left frontal brain associated with positive emotions, becomes more active as you practice meditation. The physical changes in the brain persist even weeks after practice.

With persistence and practice, you can reinforce these electrical pathways. This means that achieving a relaxation response or settling yourself down can happen more automatically as you go through your day. Similarly, you can use a simple breathing technique to activate the calming circuitry in your brain.

Practicing some form of relaxation exercise every day is a key pillar in facilitating your healing on the cancer journey. For example, some people visualize a beautiful place like a beach or a mountain meadow to generate a particular state of mind or feeling of peace and tranquility. These visualization techniques can be helpful in settling your mind and body, especially amid the stress and emotional turmoil of a cancer diagnosis. Similarly, practices like yoga and Qi Gong, with their focus on the body and the breath, can be very calming.

Benefits of Combining Relaxation Techniques with Mindfulness Meditation

Relaxation techniques are most powerful when combined with the skill of present-centered awareness that is central to mindfulness meditation. Without training in mindfulness, some people find themselves drifting back into their habitual thought patterns of worry, wishful thinking or sleepiness while engaged in a yoga pose or a visualization. Training your mind to be mindful actually increases your powers of attention to get the most benefit from many healing practices.

Mindfulness meditation is not just about feeling good for fifteen minutes while you cultivate a peaceful and present-centered state of mind. The perspective of mindfulness meditation is more vast and profound than just countering one state of mind with another. Instead of simply trying to manipulate your state of mind, you can learn to drop into the basic goodness and healthiness that is already fully present within your being.

Mindfulness Meditation and Acceptance

With mindfulness meditation, you can discover the inherent qualities in your mind such as peace, spaciousness and insight. With practice, you can learn to not only calm yourself and relax, but also to access these deeper qualities which are your essential nature and then bring them into all the activities of your daily life. Your fundamental wholesomeness is always there under the surface even if your mind is distracted and confused. It is like discovering a buried treasure that was right there all along.

The first step in uncovering our inherent wisdom with mindfulness meditation is through cultivating acceptance of 'what is'. Often our impulse in life is to turn away from the little irritations and unpleasant experiences. We distract ourselves by being busy, obsessing about the past and future, or forcing ourselves to "stay positive". This subtle tendency towards denial dulls our natural sensitivity and intelligence.

When we turn away from the truth of our experience to get lost in the familiar loops of our *thinking* mind, we lose out on the profound lessons that difficult experiences can teach us. When we do not fully pay attention to problematic patterns in our life, we can unknowingly feed the cycles that cause many painful and difficult experiences to repeat.

The simple power of mindfulness meditation is to train your mind to be present to everything in your experience as it arises, rather than to turn away. By being mindfully present to all of your experiences, feelings and thoughts as they arise, without judgment or attachment, you can gradually steady your mind, let go of problematic patterns, become aware of the moment, and cultivate spontaneous and intuitive insights.

As you confront the many challenges of a cancer diagnosis, sometimes the different voices in your mind seem to actually be engaged in conflicts with each other. For example, one thought "I want to spend more time with my family" may conflict with another thought "I need alone time to allow myself to heal." With mindful observation, you can begin to listen to these inner battles without taking sides. You can become an impartial witness to competing thoughts in some mental debate, and begin to see a clear path forward amidst your own confusion.

If you find that your mind is bouncing all over the place, like the monkey mind, just bring your mind back to the sensations in your body and your breath. This is the first step toward eventual resolution and finding the underlying wisdom in the conflict itself. You will likely experience a reprieve from conflict and worry and even realize that peace is possible in the midst of a storm.

Mindfulness meditation trains your mind to be present. When you are more present, you can begin to draw wisdom from the deep well of your wholeness which is nothing other than the fullness of life.

An Example of the Power of Meditation

Patty came to the weekend retreat having just heard that some of her test results showed that her breast cancer had spread to the lung and liver. As a nursing professor, working 80 hours a week, she felt completely out of control. She was raw emotionally, and felt like a terrible burden to her loving husband, Wally, and their two grown daughters. Her sleep was disrupted, and she felt more exhausted with each passing day. She knew chemotherapy would be coming soon but didn't even want to think about it. She was looking for tools, and a better way to 'beat the cancer.'

Like most people, Patty experienced a sense of calm when she followed the first meditation instruction on the Friday night of the retreat. Bringing her mind back to simply experiencing the sensations in her body and the act of breathing gave her a reprieve from the constant worry she had been experiencing, and a sudden realization that peace was possible in the midst of a storm.

On Friday evening, Patty told the group, "The test results showed something that I don't want to know about." Of course, she and her husband would rather not look at what the test results might mean but, at the same time, they already knew about them and this 'knowledge' was already creating anxiety for them.

In thinking about the pros and cons of the various treatment options as well as struggling with when to tell her daughters about her condition, Patty observed this inner dialogue with herself: "When do I tell my daughters? How much do I tell them? I can't bear to see them cry. I don't want to tell them. Maybe the treatments will be successful and I would worry them for nothing. I need their support now but I don't want to be a burden on them. I won't tell them until we know more. But they could come with me to the doctor's office and could be a great help in making decisions."

In her meditation Patty saw that her mind was bouncing all over the place. She found that coming back to the feeling of her body and feeling her breath gave her some moments of calm when she could face the reality of bad test results bit by bit. In facing her resistance and her fears, she felt less anxious and more willing to accept and work with her situation.

Meditation gave Patty a path to see beyond the conflicts in her mind. By gently encouraging herself to stay present to her inner battle as an impartial witness in her meditation, Patty opened up many new doors within herself where she found the courage and strength to go forward. Turning directly toward her experience, rather than turning away, allowed her to face her feelings, work through them, and make the difficult decisions about her treatments. She also realized that although she resisted telling her daughters it was the best thing to do: for them, for herself and for her husband.

CHAPTER 16

Kathy
Miracles Can Happen

"I was blindsided. How plausible could it be that I had two poten-tially fatal medical conditions fighting for supremacy in my poor, tired, bloated body? I wasn't sure whether to cry or laugh at the absurdity of this situation."

Kathy, a beautiful 47-year-old executive and mother of two teens, lay in a hospital bed recovering from the complications of a liver biopsy. Her family doctor was explaining that her Hodgkin's lymphoma (cancer of the lymph system) had recurred seven years after her first treatments. She had large masses in her chest and abdomen. In addition, for some unknown reason, her liver had been severely damaged. Her oncologist didn't want to treat her cancer because the chemotherapy would further damage her liver, and her liver specialist wouldn't recommend a liver transplant because she had active cancer. She was at a medical impasse.

Kathy knew she needed to find a way to support her body's natural capacity to heal itself so she could undergo chemotherapy. So while she would work to get her medical specialists to find a viable solution, she would also have to draw on a deep wisdom to tap into the 'power to heal.' Her inward journey started with reading the journals she had written in every night since she was a young girl.

Kathy had moved with her family from Vancouver to Hawaii when she was in her teens. Having never moved before, and leaving the familiar surroundings of her old home, she became anxious and began to worry about death and losing her mother. A mild depression ensued, providing her with a space to reflect. Her mother, who has been on a spiritual quest all her life, gave her the Bible and the writings of the Buddha. Kathy also read Edgar Cayce and stories about life after death and near-death expe-riences. She emerged from her depression with a 'knowingness' that has never left her.

Kathy later wrote "Ultimately, I somehow locked onto the notion of infinity. I thought about what was before the genesis of man. I thought about what was before that. And before that. And I realized that the human mind could not comprehend the reality of 'always was, always is.' For me, that was the defining truth: finiteness and death are a subset of infinity, of being. This did not remove the pain and hurt of mortality, but it made sense of it for me. It also gave me a feeling I can only describe as overwhelming happiness—a pervasive love and connectedness to the thing that is All."

Having this powerful spiritual insight as a young teenager gave Kathy a foundation of strength that she would later draw on throughout her life's journey. However, as often happens with such early awakenings, the glow of that peaceful joy faded and the demands of life, survival and growing up moved into the foreground.

Kathy had been painfully shy as a child, but behind her quiet persona was a fierce competitive spirit. She excelled academically and in her other activities. With a loving home environment, she was developing into a true leader. At a critical point, when her parents went through a divorce and her mother had to deal with the reality of going back to work after 25 years, Kathy vowed to herself that she would never allow herself to be dependent on others for her livelihood. This vow drove her to work hard throughout her lifetime and set in place a belief system she pushed deep within her psyche.

Pouring her spirit into the business world, she rose quickly up the corporate ladder, featured in a business magazine in her twenties as 'one to watch.' By age thirty, she was a national vice-president at a large telecommunications company. Underlying her positive and gracious persona, however, was an edge that drove her to 'outperform and outmanoeuvre her male colleagues.'

"I can see now that I was engaged in a fight that was much more about me than about 'them.' The war had been against myself. It took a lot of soul searching to see this for what it was."

By age forty, Kathy began to recognize that her life was out of balance. An increasingly stressful job forced her to contemplate her goals and what it meant to live a life of integrity. She changed jobs to align her work more closely to her heart. Then suddenly a lump developed on her neck. A biopsy showed Hodgkin's Lymphoma.

Kathy's reaction to the initial diagnosis was "Cancer? There must be a mistake." She cried in her car all the way home from the doctor's office, thinking life was unfair. But her pity party lasted a single afternoon. Her goal-oriented personality took over and she set about solving the problem of cancer much like every other challenge in her life: failure was not an option. Her mind told her she would achieve the goal, overachieve her targets, and emerge as the role model for all survivors. In an effort to be open about her diagnosis, she called a meeting of her team at work to tell them the news and was surprised to see many of them crying.

Kathy's approach to cancer was pragmatic and effective. She augmented the best conventional treatment with self-guided healing techniques, reading books such as *Love, Medicine and Miracles* by Dr. Bernie Siegel; *Anatomy of the Spirit* by Carolynn Myss; and other inspirational texts. She brushed up on her meditation and visualization skills and had reflexology sessions in her home after each chemotherapy treatment. She took vitamins, drank cleansing tea, ate all the right foods, and generally took control of the business of healing, much as she had taken control of all of the other challenges in her life.

But there was more to her journey than just getting through the treatments. Kathy began to ponder the lesson she was to take from this setback. She concluded that the cancer was a gift, sent to remind her of what was most important in life. She had two beautiful children, a great husband, and a wonderful support network of friends, family, and co-workers.

Kathy felt the cancer had been allowed to grow in her body because of the emotional turmoil, high stress, and long hours of her previous job—she comforted herself by acknowledging she had already moved into a new work role that was more in line with her true values.

After four months of chemotherapy, Kathy went back to work full time, her hair began to grow back, and she moved on with her life. Five years after her first bout with cancer, she was dismissed by her oncologist. She had achieved her goals. She believed she had emerged victorious, unscathed and convinced that she was in control of her life.

With a renewed appreciation for life, Kathy vowed to get home early and cherish her time playing with her kids and keep a happy balance. However, over the years, as the lessons from her cancer scare began to fade, she got drawn further into her work world. The prize of becoming a partner at her executive search firm tempted her to work harder and harder. In the months leading up to her recurrence of cancer, Kathy was going at an insane pace: fourteen-hour days in the office, jogging four miles to and from work with a backpack full of work clothes, calling clients from the airport before catching the red-eye to distant cities.

Her initial reaction to finding out her cancer had recurred, seven years after her original diagnosis, was, paradoxically, one of relief. In retrospect, it didn't seem surprising to her that she had become sick again. The diagnosis gave her the ultimate permission slip to jump off the treadmill again.

But with the combined diagnosis of recurrent cancer and liver damage, Kathy was trapped between two illnesses, each of which prevented treatment of the other. Despite her underlying spiritual beliefs, cancer struck fear in her heart. Leaving her kids and husband was simply not part of the plan.

Since the medical system wasn't offering any viable option, Kathy knew she had to add complementary healing, provided it was integrated with her medical treatments. She read everything she could about her two diseases, about complementary healing options, about vitamins and supplements and possible interactions with chemotherapy drugs, effects on the liver, and so on. Her research led her to a local center for integrated healing, now called InspireHealth.

She set up a full consultation with the center's co-founder, Dr. Hal Gunn, who specializes in integrative cancer care. Dr. Gunn quickly understood the medical complexities of her case and recommended a combination of vitamins and nutrition, a continued focus on fitness tailored around her treatments, and an autoimmune boosting supplement.

With the help of the medical professionals at InspireHealth, and in full collaboration with her conventional medical specialists, Kathy created a self-directed healing plan. The plan was designed to accelerate her response to chemotherapy, fortify her bodily systems to minimize damaging side effects, heal her liver, and generally improve her overall feeling of well-being. She felt empowered and involved in making herself well.

Remarkably, Kathy's liver condition stabilized enough that her medical oncologist could proceed with full-dose chemotherapy. As her physical health began to improve, her spiritual healing was just beginning. Dr. Gunn was not finished with her.

In their first session, Dr. Gunn asked why Kathy thought she had developed cancer a second time. Kathy replied that she felt she had unfinished business on the emotional and spiritual side of things. The first time she was treated for cancer, she had focused on aligning her work world with her heart. Kathy felt that this time she needed to go deeper into an understanding of why her life was still all about work. She asked herself what she was trying to prove, escape, or find?

In their next session, Dr. Gunn invited her to examine her questions further. Unable to escape the soul-connecting gaze of his clear blue eyes,

Kathy heard herself admitting a painful, hidden and core belief that she was avoiding intimacy by setting up battlegrounds both at home and at work. She needed to learn how to open her heart before she could fully heal. Her words surprised her, welling up from some buried, dark corner of her psyche.

After the appointment, the question Kathy kept asking herself was why she needed a second wakeup call. Reading her old journals, Kathy found clues to repressed insecurities she had felt most of her life that had been feeding self-doubt and a sense of inadequacy. She had compensated by developing the false persona of 'super woman'. As she sat reading her journal and reflecting on her life, she found she had to work hard to avoid judging herself. She felt she had to learn to be kind and loving toward herself.

Exposing this vulnerability left her raw and a bit emotional. By continuing to practice loving kindness and a non-judgmental attitude toward herself, however, she began to tap into a deep well of genuine compassion—for herself and for others.

Kathy discovered that practicing compassion with family members can sometimes be the most difficult challenge in life. Kathy's family culture was one of stoicism and silent strength, despite the love they felt internally. At times, Kathy interpreted her family's lack of outward signs of concern to mean that they didn't care. This led her to feel frustrated, sad and isolated. Mindful of her reactions and determined to heal these feelings of separation, Kathy began to recognize her own patterns of stoicism and to see that she had participated in creating the culture that no longer felt supportive.

Kathy realized that her self-talk was keeping her perceptions stuck in place and so she learned to reframe her thinking when she felt a family member wasn't being as supportive as she would like. The turning point for her was realizing that "It's not them, it's me. It's what I am thinking about them. I need to be able to see them for who they are. So I reframed the situation by acknowledging 'They are hurting, too. It may not show the same way that it does for me, but they need my love and compassion. They can find their heart if I open mine.'"

Years of being the strong, independent, and competitive persona had conditioned her family to give her that space which she now saw as an uncaring and distant vacuum. "They can find their heart if I open mine" was exactly the healing that her soul had prescribed.

Kathy's journey towards wholeness continued when she attended our weekend retreat. In one small group discussion, we explore the issue of death. During her first cancer diagnosis, Kathy wore the mask of the cancer heroine, never really considering that her life was at stake. When her cancer later recurred, along with advanced liver failure, she could no longer disguise the possibility of death. Kathy realized that it's not death itself that she most fears, because her reassuring insight developed as a teenager was still there within her. She knew in her heart that impermanence and death were "a subset of infinity, of being."

Although this spiritual awareness allowed her to be comfortable with the possibility of her own death, at the retreat her tears welled up as she considered its effect on her two children and husband. In a small group discussion, she shared her greatest fear: "I fear that if I don't live this moment, it could be the last. And that scares the hell out of me because I have spent most days on automatic pilot. I am busy, busy, busy. I try to do, and do some more, and then do even more. I'm focussed on achieving and making a contribution. Then my kid comes in and says, 'I need some attention', and I'm somewhere else psychologically. My greatest fear is that I'm going to miss today and that will be it. That will be the end. I will have missed out completely."

Kathy paused, brow furrowed. She stared off into a deep dark place. She was asked "What's the worst thing about dying now—from your kids' perspective?"

Kathy looked down, then back up. "That they never got to know who I was—that we didn't get underneath the veneer. They're teens now, and I'm not the fundamental part of their lives that I used to be. Will that be the memory they are left with—that I was a sick person who wasn't a friend? I don't want to be that tiny little superficial memory," Kathy was now crying openly.

In doing this deep but painful work, Kathy had lifted a shining nugget of truth from the treasure chest of her heart: that being vulnerable and looking to connect with others is her healing path. She can light her own way now with love, forgiveness, and wisdom – for herself and for others – and tap into the universal capacity to heal.

Toward the end of the retreat, Kathy shared a recent story of taking her eighteen-year-old son shopping: "I thoroughly enjoyed it. I could have been frazzled. I saw the other moms looking flustered, calling to their sons, 'Will you just get on with it? Hurry up!' My son? He's a six-foot-one 'mountain man' with washboard abs, and he comes out of the change room, does a quick turnaround, wiggles his backside at me, and asks over his shoulder with a big grin, 'Do these jeans make my butt look fat?' I just loved it. He was so cute. I just surrendered to the afternoon."

Five years after Kathy was told that her lymphoma had recurred with no viable treatment options, she now has no sign of cancer. Her oncologist says that she is a walking miracle. Her liver condition also appears stable. If Kathy needs a liver transplant, her twin sister is ready to be her donor, and the rest of her family and friends will gladly gather at her bedside to nurse her back to health.

CHAPTER 17

How to Meditate

Our minds usually jump wildly
from thought to thought.
We replay the past; we fantasize about the future.
In meditation we take an upright posture,
place our mind on an object, and keep it there.
In mindfulness meditation,
the object is the simple act of breathing.
The breath represents being alive
in the immediacy of the moment.
Sakyong Mipham

Saturday morning. The sound of chimes pierces the air. Meditation practice is about to begin. People set down their coffee cups and notebooks and assume an upright sitting position. Within seconds, an intense but peaceful energy envelops the group. Tim's voice is soft as he guides them in this meditation session.

The wonderful thing about meditation is that it includes your busy mind, your restlessness, and, in fact, all of your experience. With meditation, you cultivate a bigger mind of awareness and gentleness to work with yourself just as you are.

We do not practice meditation to become good meditators. We practice meditation to transform our lives, and to access the full potential of our humanness. If you spend five to ten minutes a day practicing, you will begin to gradually bring the increased mindfulness and awareness of meditation into your daily life.

To begin the practice of meditation, pay close attention to these three basic aspects of your life: body, breath and mind. You begin by being very attentive to your posture and your bodily sensations and then bring that same deliberate attention to the experience of breathing. Finally, bring that same mindful attention to the experience of mind.

The meditation posture here assumes that you are in a chair because that is what most people use in our retreats. However, if you prefer to sit cross-legged on a small cushion on the floor, or to kneel that is fine. You can adapt the instructions to suit your particular posture.

The meditation begins with guidance about posture, moves to following the breath, includes practice bringing the mind back to the breath, and ends with a visualization of loving kindness.

You can

(a) read this slowly to yourself or out loud;

(b) have a friend or family member read it out loud for you; or

(c) listen to it for free on an audio file available at
     www.healingandcancer.org

If you or someone else is reading it, proceed very slowly, pausing at each line, and taking the time to follow the instructions as they come.

Enjoy this journey…

Sitting in your chair feel the weight of your body
*   pressing against the seat*
Place your feet flat on the floor and feel the sensations there
Feel what it is like to make contact with the floor below
Rest your hands gently on your knees or thighs
Feel the sensations of contact there in your hands and legs
Tune into your body, feel the sensations in your body
Notice whatever part of your body calls, then listen
Feel your connection to gravity, your connection to the energy
*   of the earth below*
Now lean a little further forward to arch the lumbar spine slightly
Then come back up straight
Take an upright and dignified posture in the chair
Keeping a little arch in the lower back to lift you up a bit
Your lower body is solid and grounded to the earth
Your upper body and spine are rising upwards out of the pelvis
Now open up your heart and chest area
By lifting your chest up and forward, just a tiny bit

Now feel the crown of your head
Feel as if it were being pulled up, gently, by a string
As if there were a string coming down from the sky
Gently pulling at the very top of your head
This will bring you to tuck your chin just a little bit
So the back of your neck is long

Now that you have a nice straight spine
Let yourself completely relax on that structure
Relax your belly, relax your shoulders, relax everywhere
Let your spine support you, let go of all tension
Just as the structure of a building needs no muscles to hold it up
You can relax on the structure of your spine and
   the structure of your bones
Let it hold you up straight and natural, easily balanced without effort
You can leave your eyes open, if you like, resting downward
Three to six feet ahead on the floor in front of you
With eyes open, you stay awake and alert in your meditation,
If you need to, you can briefly close your eyes to rest them
Staying mindful and alert to the sensations in your body
Lastly, you can also rest your tongue on the upper palette
Just behind your upper teeth
This connects an important energy loop in the body
And gives your tongue a place to be still and quiet

Now bring your attention to your breathing
See if you can feel the breath in your nostrils,
In your throat, in your lungs
Feel the muscles that go to work on the in-breath
And feel them relax on the out breath
Be present to the sensations of the in breath
And present to the sensations of the out-breath
Breathing in… and out… is the rhythm of life
Expansion…contraction,
Receiving… giving
See if you can breathe down into the lower abdomen just a bit
Breathe down into your belly
Then as you breathe out, let your attention go out as well

Allow yourself to relax with the outgoing breath
As you breathe out, relax and let go
Let your mindful attention dissolve with the breath as it goes out
Tune into your body and presence as you breathe in
Honouring this good body, not taking it for granted
If you're here and breathing
Then there are a million things working right with your body
And you can celebrate that right here and right now
With each breath celebrate the life energy that
    courses through your body
Do you notice a sense of aliveness
Honour your aliveness, here in this present moment
Feel the earth below supporting you
A sense of firmness and solidity grounding you here and now
Then feel the fluid moving and spaciousness of the breath

If your mind wanders off into thinking about something else,
bring it gently back to this very moment
Bring your attention back to the breath
And back to the sensations in your body
Come back to the sensation of being here breathing
Come back to the actual sensation of each breath as you breathe it

If there's a feeling of restlessness or irritation
Just acknowledge that
Normally through the day we keep ourselves so busy
Now in this silence and stillness of meditation
That engine of busyness may still be running
There is a lot of busyness momentum there
It has been built up over your entire life
Try to breathe into that restless, busy momentum and soften to it
Let go with the out-breath, expand into space
Make friends with that feeling of restlessness and let it be
Let it unwind itself in the space of your breath
Sometimes we call this restlessness 'anxiety' or 'worry'
For now let's just investigate that energy carefully
Without judging it, without labelling it
Just be present to that raw energy of restlessness

Because that is your life energy
And it has a tremendous healing power
Hidden within it

As you work to be mindful of each breath
Sometimes thoughts will pull your mind away
As soon as you notice that
Simply bring your attention back to breathing
Back to being present in your body
Present to feeling body
Present to feeling breath

Each time you notice that your attention has strayed from the breath
Strayed from being present, here and now,
Whenever attention is pulled completely into thoughts
You can actually label those thoughts as "thinking"
Simply say silently to yourself, "thinking"
At this very moment,
Then let go of the thought
And come back to the experience of breathing

By labelling your thoughts in this way
You gradually grow wise to that moment of waking up
That moment of being awake to the here and now

Notice that thoughts will come and go
It is the nature of your mind to give rise to thoughts
That is not a problem
You don't need to get rid of your thoughts

Thoughts come and go like puffy clouds in a clear blue sky
The clouds shift, move and change and then they dissipate,
They dissolve back into their nature
Which is the openness of the clear blue sky
If you find yourself off on a cloud, lost in thinking
Simply say to yourself, "thinking"
Then gently bring your attention back to your breathing
Back to your presence

Back to feeling the life force pulsing in your body
Enjoy the feeling of being alive, breathing, awake and present

Now you will do a brief meditation and visualization of loving kindness
To begin this tune into your own good human heart
There is your physical heart on the left side
And then there is your energetic heart center
In the middle of your chest
Tune into that energetic heart center
And let it warm up just like turning on a burner on the stove
It begins to glow with radiant warmth
Merely by bringing your attention here
You can begin to ignite the fires of loving kindness
If you like, you can think of someone you love
Think of someone you love very much and send them that love
Notice how that feels
There is a subtle sensation
The natural radiant love shines out from your heart
Now send that loving light to every cell of your body
Every part of your being
Loving yourself exactly as you are here and now
Flood your body with this healing light
This is the energy of loving kindness
It is always there, always available
When you bring your attention to it
When you remember it, you cultivate it, you enhance it
You can enhance this good loving heart with your attention
You can use it to heal
Use it to reclaim your already existing wholeness
And to connect with others in the wholeness of our healing circle
Allow your heart to open and radiate
As if your heart was the shining sun itself
Radiating the light of loving kindness
Love yourself and heal back into wholeness

Letting go now of the image of radiant love
Letting go of the practice of loving kindness
Come back to being fully present

Come back to basic mindfulness meditation
Feel each breath again just as it is
Relax and let go as you breathe out
Mindful of body
Mindful of breath
Connect now with the space around you
Maintain this sense of being present
Awake and aware here and now
With an open heart
As you go forward into life

You might find that there is a lot to coordinate here to follow the instructions fully. The first time you do anything it can feel awkward or difficult. This is not a problem in the least.

When people are first learning to meditate on the weekend retreats, some will seem restless, shifting uncomfortably in their chairs. Others will tell us "I just couldn't settle." Or even "I couldn't meditate because my mind was so busy." This is a normal reaction when people first learn to meditate. That is why we call it a practice. Meditation requires consistent effort over an extended time.

You may have a profound experience one time and then feel completely distracted and unfocussed with a "monkey mind" the next. This is a normal and natural experience of meditation practice. What matters is making the effort and following the instructions consistently. Gradually, over time, meditation begins to work on you.

Many people are hard on themselves and are driven to be perfect. Meditation is learning to make friends with yourself. When you befriend someone, you learn to listen with patience and a non-judgmental attitude. With time you develop a deep appreciation for your friend. With meditation, you can cultivate this loving-kindness towards yourself.

CHAPTER 18

My Meditation Practice

Deep peace on the running wave to you
Deep peace on the flowing air to you
Deep peace on the quiet earth to you
Deep peace of the shining stars to you
Deep peace on the gentle night to you
Moon and stars pour their healing light on you
Deep peace to you
Traditional Gaelic Blessing

Saturday morning. Rob shares the experience of his daily meditation practice to show that meditation is not mystical or otherworldly and that meditating has been helpful in his life as an oncologist.

Over a decade ago Tim taught me how to meditate. Most mornings I get up forty minutes earlier than I would have otherwise, go downstairs to my meditation area, kneel down on a couple of pillows and assume a straight and comfortable posture. I bring my attention to my breathing and the sensations of my body. Typically, about two seconds after starting, my mind starts to drift off and I begin to think about something else. Usually I start planning what I need to do that day: the jobs that have to get done, the people I need to talk to, what I will say at a particular meeting. At some point, sometimes minutes later, I realize that I am thinking about the future and not mindfully attending to my breath or my body. Noticing this, without judgment, I simply bring my attention back to my breath.

A few seconds later my chattering mind starts up again. I might think about what happened the previous day: what I should have said in a particular conversation, how guilty or embarrassed I felt about my actions. I replay these scenes in my mind thinking about alternate endings. Eventually I realize I'm thinking about the past and not focusing on the present. Again I'm very gentle on myself and I bring my attention back to breathing. Back and forth it goes – dozens of times within that forty minutes: I'm mindfully focused on breathing, I'm off thinking, I'm mindfully focused again, I'm off thinking......

Sometimes at about the thirty minute point, something snaps in me and suddenly I feel like I'm sinking into my body right in the here and now. I can experience a deep feeling of peace, relaxation and spaciousness

Interestingly, my chattering mind does not stop chattering at that point. In some way though, it seems not to chat so loudly, or perhaps, I am less concerned and less invested in the dramas of my own thoughts. Then I feel generally more present, even though the thoughts still come and go.

On the days when I do meditate in the morning I feel more peaceful and grounded throughout my day. I am better able to listen to the person in front of me in the cancer centre and at home with my family. My innate caring and compassion comes out more when I meditate regularly.

Meditating makes me a better doctor and, paradoxically, despite feeling calm and relaxed, I'm much more efficient. I do one thing at a time and my day seems to flow more easily. I can focus on the details as well as see the bigger picture, including how my emotions rise and fall without being caught up in them.

Over the years not much has changed as I practice each morning. Some mornings, I settle into being present sooner and I'm better able to see the thoughts coming and going undisturbed. Other mornings, I get taken off on long stories in my mind and remain agitated. But whether the experience of meditation goes well or not, I keep coming back to it.

A few years ago, I realized that I was practicing the same skill of mindfulness meditation throughout the day. As I was talking to someone I would catch myself thinking about something else completely. I wasn't paying attention to the person or what was happening in the situation. In the same way that I bring my attention back to my breathing during the morning meditation, I would simply refocus my attention on the person and the situation. The same sequence of being caught up in my mind, thinking of something else, realizing it, then re-focusing on the moment, happens all day long.

With practice I am remaining more in the present throughout my life. I am better able to pay attention to my body, receiving its feedback so I can take better care of myself. I'm more in touch with my emotions so that they are less likely to negatively influence how I treat others. And meditation has allowed me to see that my thoughts come and go. I am better able to let them just be, without getting caught up in strategies for their future or reliving new versions of stories from the past.

Meditation has made me a better person. I am forever more grateful to Tim for teaching me to be kind to myself and to recognize my own wholeness.

CHAPTER 19

Talking about Stress

Be patient to all that is unsolved in your heart,
And try to love the questions themselves.
Do not seek the answers that cannot be given you,
Because the point is to live everything,
Live the questions now.
Perhaps you will gradually without noticing it,
Live along some distant day into the answers.
Rainer Maria Rilke

Saturday morning. *After finishing a short meditation, the people in the healing circle appear relaxed as they leave the large group and gather into small groups of six or seven for discussion. Their faces are calm and their shoulders appear to have softened.*

Drawing on his knowledge of the physiology of stress, Rob begins by asking his small group to identify their stressors, and their unique stress reaction.

When was the last time you felt suddenly stressed, scared, angry or upset? Think about situations in which you were super stressed. They could be related to the cancer diagnosis, like going in for a medical appointment, or anything else in your life, like work or with your family.

As you recall your stress reaction, imagine a computer could measure every sensation in your body you were experiencing, every emotion you felt and every thought going through your mind. What the computer would sense is your unique physical and emotional reaction to stress. Or another way to ask it is 'How do your body and emotions let you know when you are stressed?'

Nancy is the first to speak. She's a 50-year-old woman who lost her job as a manager in a massive restructuring just before her diagnosis of fallopian tube cancer. Recovering from a major operation and six months of chemotherapy, and living alone, she's in the midst of trying to rebuild her life. Her voice becomes thin as she recounts her experience of going into an operating room for the first time in her life. Just before the operation, her physician told her that he couldn't see enough from the CAT scan to know what he would find when he 'opened her up.' "The nurses were tying my arms down to the operating table while they were getting me to sign the consent form. I felt so out of control. It was all so stressful."

After a lifetime of working hard, planning her life step by step, the loss of control is very hard on Nancy. "Will the cancer recur? Will I get through the operation? Will I need chemotherapy? What are the side effects? How can I afford being off work? What am I going to do!!!??"

Nancy pauses, and then reflects on the question about her physical symptoms of stress. "When I feel this stressed, my body goes into high speed tension. I'm shaking inside. I start pacing."

Stress experts Lazarus and Folman defined the stress reaction as a condition in which an individual perceives the demands of the situation as exceeding their resources. When Nancy perceives that she is not in total control of her life (and believes she should be), this initiates a chemical reaction in the primitive part of her brain that releases adrenaline, the 'fight or flight' hormone, into her blood stream.

Adrenaline gives her body a sudden burst of energy. It causes Nancy's heart to pump hard and fast. Her blood pressure goes up. She takes quick shallow breaths high in her chest. Her digestive tract shuts down, causing symptoms of an acidy stomach, complete with cramps or "butterflies", and her blood is sent to increasingly tense muscles, causing pain or jitters. Adrenaline causes a sense of panic, headache, sweaty palms, and other disturbing symptoms.

The second major hormone released during the stress reaction is cortisol, which increases the sugars and fats in the blood. Every time Nancy feels overwhelmed, adrenaline and cortisol bathe every cell in her body.

Unfortunately, frequent stress reactions suppress Nancy's body's natural ability to heal. Stress hormones break down body tissue, including the very DNA that instructs every cell how to do its work. The stress reaction suppresses the immune system, which, in a more relaxed state, can help fight off cancer cells and infections. If Nancy continues to live in a high-strung state, she'll be susceptible to heart attacks, diabetes, inflammation like arthritis, ulcers, chronic pain, and dementia…just to list a few.

Kathy, an executive recovering from Hodgkin's Lymphoma and auto-immune liver disease, identifies anger as her response to stressful situations. "If someone treats me with disrespect, like some woman tries to butt in front of me in line, I just go crazy. I get really angry. I feel like I have to defend myself." She notices the stress reaction in her body as a constriction in her throat, so much so that sometimes she feels like she can't speak.

Kathy is mindful of her body's reaction to feeling stressed and can begin 'de-stressing' before she gets too worked up. Her flash of anger illustrates that the stress reaction includes an emotional reaction that even changes how she thinks. She becomes irritated, emotional, angry and ready to act. She is primed to fight or flee, often without being able to think through the problem.

Bonnie, a breast cancer survivor, now in her seventies, pipes up. She has had a lifetime full of looking after others. She sacrificed her own needs when her husband went back to school to get a Ph.D. She cared for their children almost single-handedly and really ran all aspects of the household, including the finances. The pattern continued as her husband invested more of his time in his work. Sadly, upon retirement, he was diagnosed with multiple myeloma, and Bonnie was his primary caregiver through the last seven years of his life.

Now that he's gone, his absence contributes to her feeling of emptiness which also causes stress. "When you're in a loving relationship for a long time and accustomed to doing everything together, it's stressful to do things on your own. Now I have to go to tests and cancer doctors by myself and nobody is there to go back home to."

When asked to identify a stressful situation, Bonnie talks about all the responsibilities of homeownership, including suddenly dealing with an "exploding" toilet. Having to get the maintenance man in, and dealing with several problems all at the same time, was very stressful. When she's stressed Bonnie feels tension in her back, and her gut goes into knots.

But like many people, Bonnie has a hard time recognizing her own stress reaction because she has always focused outwardly, always has been the one to wrap the blanket of care around others. So, in a demanding situation, she tends to disconnect from her body and its needs. She doesn't connect the back tension with her stress. Instead she focuses on taking care of problems—mostly everyone else's. She ends up not paying attention to her body's messages and pushes herself beyond her limits.

The aching gut and the tension in her back may be the only signals telling Bonnie 'This is too much. I need your attention.' If Bonnie listens mindfully to her internal signs of stress, she can then take better care of herself and be more effective in the outer world.

Liz, a lady in her mid fifties tells the group "I feel a lot of stress from being disrespected, having people try to mould me the way they prefer. I don't like the pressure of other people's expectations."

Liz worked as a teacher, often choosing to work in inner city schools where many of the children needed her loving attention. She was first diagnosed with a rare carcinoid tumor of the lung ten years ago which was treated easily with an operation. Then, a year ago, she began to notice a pain in her hip which happened just at the same time her personal physician moved away. She went to her husband's doctor but says "I don't feel comfortable with him. He shuts me down. He doesn't take me seriously. I spent a year trying to talk to him but I was always cut off and told 'It's just arthritis'.

"I never show my frustration when I'm in that kind of situation. I hide my stress. I've always done that. It's just like when I was a teen at the dinner table. I was saying to my Dad 'I'm going to university.' He said, 'Huh, I'll believe that when I see it.' I just got quiet and didn't say anything. It's one thing to deal with the cancer coming back in my hip but worse when I can see that I fall back into being how I was in my family, when I was young."

Liz was very angry with the delay in the diagnosis because the doctor hadn't listened to her and she spent several days crying, blaming others, and thinking how stupid the doctor was. "Gradually I settled down and got myself back into nightly meditation and my usual healing yoga routine. And things started to calm down."

Liz returns to the question of where in her body she experiences stress. "When I'm upset I feel a constriction in my third eye," she points to her forehead between her eyes. "I feel this swelling, sometimes to the point of bursting. In every picture from my childhood, I'm frowning there."

Not only were the sensations on Liz's forehead raising a red flag of stress – they were also providing a gateway to unresolved issues she had long kept inside. It was only by paying attention to the physical clues that she was able to make these deeper associations. She realized that not all of her anger was coming from thinking about the delays caused by her physician. Old emotions from not being taken seriously long ago were coming to the surface. Through awareness she began to heal these psychological issues.

Jan speaks next. In her early fifties, she continues to struggle with the long-term effects of her rectal cancer which occurred seven years earlier. Her gut is unreliable, forcing her to run off to the bathroom at a moment's notice. Feeling stressed makes this worse. Her job is stressful and she feels her workplace is broken. She wonders whether to quit now or try to make it to retirement.

But mostly Jan worries about her family and the myriad of other people in her life. A few years ago, her adult daughter survived a terrible accident. Starting in the months that followed the accident, albeit less so recently, Jan sometimes feels an "instant jolt of anxiety", like a huge wave starting in her stomach and rolling up her chest, sometimes sticking in her throat.

This anxiety can hit her just from seeing her daughter's name come up on the call screener. When she's too upset she simply does not answer the phone. Later, when she notices that her body has settled, she plays the answering machine message and calls her daughter back from a position of peace and true love. Jan wisely knows her own limits and how she can best use her precious energy.

Jan listens to the wisdom of her body to guide her towards healing and contentment. Instead of focusing solely on the 'negative' messages from her body, she also notices when she feels good. "When I'm on the right track, making the decisions that are right for me, I get this feeling in my body of being grounded. I feel my energy even in my legs. I've got bounce. And my chest feels light and starts to hum." She feels a deep calm in her gut and her mind remains open and clear. By working through her emotional blocks and following the positive sensations from her body, Jan is moving forward on her journey towards wholeness.

Antidotes to Stress

The last few minutes of the small group discussion focus on what people do to help themselves when they recognize their own stress reaction.

Kathy says she pauses and takes a few slow breaths deep into my belly. She also adds a variation to this classic relaxation technique: "When I breathe, I smile. It makes me feel like laughing."

Working the smiling muscles actually energizes the very part of Kathy's brain responsible for laughing. She can catch a quick updraft of emotion simply by smiling, lifting up her cheeks, squinting her eyes, and chuckling at herself. Like the relaxation breath, smiling actually changes the chemicals in her brain and body.

Kathy describes how she deals with situations such as someone cutting in front of her in line. "Now I use compassion in the situation. When my ego is feeling thwarted, I look for the beauty in the other person. I think 'That person is having a worse day than I am.' This helps my soul."

Jan, who took care of everyone in her family, including her husband during his seven-year cancer journey, uses a simple Christian prayer to find her inherent resilience and compassion: "Thy will be done." She acknowledges she doesn't have full control over the situation and, beyond doing what she can, is willing to let God choose the outcome.

Nancy uses the energy of feeling stressed to do constructive things for herself. When she's feeling hyped up for any reason, she not only works with the source of the stress, but also takes that energy right into an exercise routine or something else physical like pushing a lawnmower.

Nancy says she feels great after a workout, and, while exercising, has time to reflect and gain perspective. While tending to be practical in her response to stress, she also taps into deeper inner resources. She shares a quote from a friend: "What lies behind us and what lies before us are tiny matters compared to what lies within us." She adds, "That brings me back to where I am."

CHAPTER 20

Practicing the Relaxation Response in the Chaos of Life

The natural healing force within each of us is the greatest force in getting well.
Hippocrates

Saturday morning. One of the most stressful experiences people at the retreats describe is going to their doctors to get test results. Rob tells the story of seeing some of his patients shaking in their chairs with worry about what he might say. He feels badly and wants to offer them something they can do to settle themselves — without prescribing a sedative.

At the weekend retreat, Rob teaches a simple and powerful relaxation exercise and he explains how this technique can be applied in daily life when faced with sudden stressful situations in their lives.

Fifty people stand in a large circle and, on cue, pretend they have just been suddenly frightened. Rob shouts "BOO" and in a single spasm, shoulders hunch, eyes widen, foreheads furrow, and the sound of one quick inhalation fills the room.

Rob continues. "You can really feel yourself start to get worked up. Now relax. Let go of the tension in your body. Put one hand on your abdomen and the other on your chest. As you breathe slowly let your breath drop down deep into your belly, and allow your chest to soften."

Being able to identify your unique stress reaction is the first crucial step in reversing the harmful effects of acute stress. Through ongoing mindfulness of the sensations in your body, emotional reactions, and thinking, you can gradually become wise to your unique stress reaction. As you become more aware of the repeating patterns, you can start to choose how to react to the situations which trigger your stress reaction and the underlying beliefs which cause the upset.

As well, the earlier you identify the initial symptoms of what will lead to feeling panicked, angry, or overwhelmed, the easier it will be to change the energy and to return to a healthier and happier state. It takes practice and an ongoing commitment to really pay attention to what is happening in your life, both in your inner and outer worlds. But, with experience, you gain insight into how to "de-stress" when you see yourself getting worked up.

As soon as you identify that you're beginning to feel stressed, you can use the following four steps of the 'belly breathing' technique to develop a relaxation response to a stressful situation:

1 *Pause:* Press the 'pause' button. Let go of trying to do something right away until you look at the situation closely. This non-action phase usually works well because there are very few situations in which you must act immediately.

2 *Pay attention:* Be curious about what you are feeling. Really slow down in that moment and carefully watch your reactions as if for the very first time, and as if you are outside yourself. Watching includes being aware of your physical sensations, your emotions and the thoughts that go through your mind. For example, ask yourself: "What exactly does that sore muscle feel like? Are my butterflies in the upper or lower abdomen? Are there more butterflies this time than last? What sensations are telling me that my heart is beating harder?"

Being mindful of what's happening in your body automatically engages the part of your brain responsible for relaxation and insight. The electrical activity in the primitive brain becomes less active and the part of your brain that is creative and good at problem solving becomes more active. This physiological change may enable you to think of new or appropriate approaches to the situation.

Shifting the attention from the outside world to your inner responses also primes your body for the 'breathing' part of the 'belly breathing' technique.

3 *Breathe:* Breathe deeply into your belly. Take a long, slow breath deep into your pelvis to initiate a sense of calm and peacefulness. Bring your mindfulness to all of the bodily sensations of this breath, such as feeling air going through your nose and the sensations of your abdomen rising.

Repeat this same slow breath three or four times, with each breath focusing more and more on your body. This anti-stress breath taps into the relaxation response which allows you to feel calmer.

4 *Talk to yourself:* Be kind and encourage yourself to find a place of greater calm, peace and clarity. Use a kind and wise voice in your mind to say something like "I will have the strength to face whatever happens." or "I can bring love and peace to any situation."

By practicing this 'breathing' technique in stressful situations you will notice that you can settle yourself down more quickly. The effectiveness of this technique increases even more if you practice some type of relaxation technique every day when you're not stressed. The circuitry of the relaxation response gets more deeply engrained with time and your ability to 'remember' that feeling will improve.

Be Kind to Yourself

If you're hard on yourself for feeling stressed when you think you shouldn't be, then you may be contributing further to your stress reaction. This 'de-stressing' or 'relaxation response' technique will not make all the stressful situations in your life go away. Whether it's on a cancer journey, at work or at home, you will continue to face challenges throughout your life. It's part of being human and living a full life.

By applying mindfulness in everyday life you can wake up to both the causes and effects of stress. By practicing belly breathing when you need it, you will gradually decrease your physiological stress and the symptoms it causes. Gradually as stress diminishes, you'll find you can reorient yourself in your life to become more content, clearer about who you are, and what your priorities are. All this will help you relax into the chaos of everyday life.

CHAPTER 21

Pam
Just Being Me

"I didn't ever feel like I got the love that I needed growing up. Being the third child of four, there weren't even any pictures of me as a baby. I used to run away from home a lot, then eventually turn around and come back, feeling like nobody really cared whether I was there or not."

Sitting in our afternoon discussion group at the retreat, Pam's eyes shine out brightly under the dark turban on her head. She speaks of the great pain in her 53 years with tenderness, warmth and a knowing smile, suggesting she had been through an extraordinary transformation.

Though her childhood was often painful, Pam was determined to make a difference in the lives of others. Trained as a social worker at university, she took a job in a state-run mental hospital and, years later, in a large cancer centre. In both of these positions, she found herself buried under a huge caseload and rarely had time to give each patient or family member the attention she knew they needed and deserved. These pressures eventually led to burnout and, in time, she sought less demanding work.

She often fell into depression and isolation, and walked away from two unhealthy relationships. Suffering from suicidal thinking, she periodically took time off to deal with her own mental health and rebalance her life. In the midst of these struggles, she had the inspiration to become a mother so that she could experience giving and receiving unconditional love without holding back. Her family doctor, also a friend, told her that she had so much love to give and agreed Pam would be a wonderful mother. Using an agency to obtain an anonymous sperm sample, Pam became pregnant, and within a couple of years had two 'miracle' children.

Pam's eyes beam with joy when she thinks back to those years. It was a hard time financially and emotionally, but she had a steady, low-stress job working at home and could devote all of her energy to raising her children in a loving environment.

As her kids reached their teens, her lifelong struggle of not being able to appreciate and truly love herself continued. "I was doing my best to meet the challenges, and often received praise from others for my work, but I couldn't appreciate myself at all. In the back of my mind, I was always looking for an exit strategy, a way out. There wasn't a lot pulling me to life, other than wanting to be there for my children."

Pam looks down, contemplating the years in her life that seemed to drag on and on after her kids became independent. Her grandmother became sick, then an uncle, then her mother became frail. Every time someone needed her, she would dedicate herself graciously to help them however she could.

However, feelings of being unworthy simmered underneath her pleasant disposition. "When you believe that you are not really wanted or loved, you do everything you can to prove that you are worthy and good, but as long as that root belief is under there, it really doesn't work." The never ending treadmill of constant service to others without loving herself was taking its toll. A persistent thought plagued Pam that strangely foreshadowed what was to come: "Wouldn't it be convenient to get a terminal illness?"

There is a calm acceptance in how she tells the rest of her story. The month after the last ailing relative died, Pam decided, uncharacteristically, to do something for herself. She decided to treat herself to a trip to Greece, but a pre-travel X-ray showed a shadow in her lungs and the biopsy confirmed advanced lung cancer. Pam was shocked.

Her oncologist told her that without treatment she'd have about two months to live. Pam's response was visceral, "Oh my god! That's not enough time!" She had waited all those years, taking care of others, and was finally trying to enjoy her own life now. She quickly accepted the offer of chemotherapy.

She remembers a day when she was in hospital that her daughter Kathryn was there, playing a lute, serenading Pam with heavenly music and her loving presence. Pam's heart swells remembering the words of advice from her twenty-year-old confidante: "Mom, this cancer is a blessing. This is your life. This is your opportunity to really live."

Pam's whole face brightens. "That stirred me more than anything else. My daughter has such insight and enthusiasm, and this is the child that's going to be left without a mother. But I knew she was right. I could see the really tight timeline in the future as a blessing. I felt it is now or never for me to do everything I want to do in life."

Pam's voice begins to strengthen and a new confidence takes over her being as she describes the many ways she has chosen to nurture herself and reclaim her spirit. She read an inspiring book by Louise Hay called *You Can Heal Your Life*. In it she learned that affirmations can be a powerful way to focus on healing psychological wounds and setting an intention to heal. The affirmation the author suggested for people with cancer was 'I lovingly forgive and release all my past. I chose to fill my life with joy. I love and approve of myself.' She learned it by heart and recited it frequently while walking down the street and while digging her fingers into the soil of her garden.

She found herself smiling and noticing people. Lights seemed to change when she wanted to cross the street. It seemed like the world was really opening up and receiving her. She couldn't explain what was happening, but these coincidences reinforced a sense that she was on the right path and opening to a divine presence. A different set of thoughts came to mind: 'If I can be cured, great. If I can't, then it is still going to be a good ride, a chance to heal and reclaim my spirit.'

Pam was drawn to the Healing Journey program developed by Dr. Alastair Cunningham, available as a home study course. One exercise asked her to vividly imagine what her life will be like in three years. The question intrigued her because none of the doctors had given her three years to live.

Imagining what the ideal morning would be like in the future, she pictured walking in the woods, writing in her journal, watching the sun rise and practicing Tai Chi. She then realized that she could do all these same things in the present, and began walking through the park early every morning. She followed the routine but mostly she just 'flowed' with whatever was happening. Walking home from this daily practice she felt energized and prepared for the day.

Pam's eyes glow as she looks to the group. "My daughter was right. My cancer diagnosis has been a gift. It has given me time to learn to be myself. I've had a lot more joy in the last nine months than I have had in my whole life. I have released tons of negative things from my outer life and from inside myself. I am not driven by that image of who I think I should be any more. Just being me is a lovely and comfortable place to be."

Reframing
Distressing Thoughts

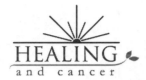

HEALING
and cancer

Saturday afternoon • Reframing Distressing Thoughts

In this section of the book, you will learn how to 'reframe' distressing thoughts by reviewing multiple real-life examples, listening to lectures and stories, and joining the small and large groups as the participants discuss their most upsetting issues.

Reframing distressing thoughts, using the simple three-column technique taught here, helps you draw on your innate wisdom and kindness, and develop a different perspective of the difficult situations that arise on the cancer journey. The weekend teachings uniquely integrate modern psychology, loving-kindness and the ancient practice of mindfulness.

The skill of reframing, practiced with love for yourself and others, can have a transformative and healing effect on all aspects of your life.

CHAPTER 22

"Tell Me About the Place You Come From"

*Only in growth, reform and change,
paradoxically enough,
is true security to be found.*
Anne Morrow Lindbergh

Saturday afternoon. *After moving through a Chinese energy exercise called Qi Gong, the people at the retreat settle into their chairs in a circle to listen to Tim tell a story.*

A long time ago in a time that is beyond time, there was a pleasant little village in the country with a rock wall around it and a little gate near the road where people came into the village from the countryside.

On a bench by the gate sat an old wise man. He liked to sit still and look out over the fields. On a lovely spring day he looked down the road and beyond through the fields to the woods and into the distance. He looked out just to see whatever came up.

On this day, after a quiet morning, along came a young man who seemed to be in search of something. He was walking down the road with determination, but seemed lost in his thoughts, looking down and kicking at the ground every now and then. He stopped at the gate and addressed the elderly fellow, "Tell me, old man, what's this village like? What are the people like? Would this be a good place to settle down and raise a family?"

The old man looked at him carefully for a while and then said, "Well, tell me about the place where you come from. What's that like?"

"That town!" exclaimed the young man. "I hate that town. I don't feel comfortable there. People are not very nice to each other. There is a lot of arguing and conflicts and frustration. Nobody understands me there. I am fed up with that place; that's why I left."

The old man at the gate nodded while he listened, then after a while said, "Well, you know, you might find this village to be a lot like the one you just left."

"Well, if that's true," said the younger man, "Then I'm moving on and I'm going to find another place." So he marched right through the little village, hardly noticing anything about it, and kept on searching.

A little while later another young fellow came walking down the road. He was looking up, enjoying the birds and the wind blowing through the grasses on this fresh spring day. As he approached the wise old man, he too asked, "Tell me, what's this village like? What are the people like? Is it a nice place to settle down and raise a family?"

Again the old man paused and looked at him carefully, then asked, "Well, tell me about the place where you come from. What's that like?"

"Oh, it's a lovely place, a wonderful place. Our village is prosperous and the people are generally happy. We try to be kind to one another." Then he paused to think for a minute. "Everybody is very special there, very different from one another. We like it that way. We appreciate the differences in each person. We try to get along and we are kind to one another. When people are sick or unhappy we surround them with loving attention. My family and friends were very kind to me there. I loved it but I have come exploring, seeking my fortune, and I just wondered if this village would be a nice place to settle down."

The old man at the gate nodded and said, "Well, you know, you might find this village to be a lot like the one you just left."

Tim is silent to mark the end of the story. "What's happening here?" He asks.

Someone shouts, "<u>You</u> are the village!" Another calls out "Wherever You Go, There You Are" which is the title to one of Jon Kabat-Zinn's books. Finally, a wise old woman calls out from the back, "Your attitude and perspective determine how you experience the world."

"Yes." Tim responds enthusiastically. "We bring our own attitudes and our own perspectives into every situation. We project these onto each situation. Then the situation begins to absorb whatever it is that we project onto it and feed it back to us. It is almost like the world is a blank screen and our minds are the movie projectors."

Tim pauses, and then asks "How is it that we tend to carry the past into the present, and even project it onto the future? What is the mechanism?"

Again, the woman in the back says "with our thoughts."

"Yes!" responds Tim, "And that is why it is so important to be mindful of our thoughts and to start noticing how our thoughts tend to shape our experience of life. But we have a choice about what we think. We can develop skills to 'reframe distressing thoughts' and change them with mindfulness, insight, and kindness."

CHAPTER 23

Reframing "I can't do it"
A Practical Exercise

We are upset not by things
but the view we take of them
Epictetus

Saturday afternoon. Reframing distressing thoughts is a practice that helps you begin to see repeating patterns in your life and the interconnection between your thoughts and emotions. To start, you need to learn to cultivate mindfulness of your thoughts themselves, with a non-judgmental attitude, and begin to recognize the distorted thoughts that tend to create emotional turmoil. Ultimately, by reframing distressing thoughts, you can reduce your stress and despair, and rest more often in your natural state of calm and compassion.

Tim begins his lecture pointing to the three-column table up on the screen.

Mindful of Distressing and Automatic Thoughts	Inquiry and Insight	Kind and Rational Response
	• What emotions follow this way of thinking? • Is this a helpful or harmful thought? • Is this thought exaggerated or irrational?	

The three column technique for reframing distressing thoughts is based on the work of Dr. David Burns, a psychiatrist who wrote the classic book 'Feeling Good'. Dr. Burns shows that distorted thinking patterns can actually cause you to feel depressed and anxious, and that when you train yourself to think more clearly in a rational and realistic way, you will experience greater self-esteem, and more joy and intimacy in your relationships.

More recently this psychological approach has been combined with the ancient practice of mindfulness into 'mindfulness-based cognitive therapy'. This therapy has been proven effective in many different conditions, and modern neuroscience shows that the pathways and activity in your brain actually change when you teach yourself to reframe distressing thoughts.

It's easiest to learn this technique by taking real-life situations and examining how your thoughts affect your emotions, and how to view the situation from a wiser and more compassionate perspective.

The following example is based on a situation in which someone, going through chemotherapy, is physically tired and emotionally raw. In addition to the truth of the situation, the person thinks to himself or herself "It's no use. I don't have the strength to get through this."

In the left column in the table below, under the heading 'Mindful of Distressing and Automatic Thoughts,' the person would write down their distressing thought:

Mindful of Distressing and Automatic Thoughts	Inquiry and Insight	Kind and Rational Response
"It's no use. I don't have the strength to get through this."	• What emotions follow this way of thinking? • Is this a helpful or harmful thought? • Is this thought exaggerated or irrational?	

The *first step* in reframing is to be mindful of a particular distressing thought (left column). By writing it down, it is easier to recognize what we have been saying to ourselves. The *second step* (middle column) is to investigate this thought carefully by asking ourselves what emotions follow from this way of thinking, whether the thought is helpful or harmful, and in what ways the thought may be exaggerated or irrational. The *third step* (right column) is to use a kind and rational approach to reframe the thought.

Tim asks the group to reflect on the question: 'How is the thought separate from the situation?' Tim explains "The *situation* is that the person is very tired, they have suffered side effects of treatment and they are feeling depressed and upset. The *thought* 'It's no use. I don't have the strength to get through this' is extra. It's a conclusion, and it causes additional suffering. When we see that thought coming up and realize it is not helping, we can actually start working with the thought itself."

So next Tim invites the group to consider the questions in the middle column, under the title "Inquiry and Insight." He asks: "What sorts of emotions follow from this way of thinking?" The group comes to life. A flurry of single-word answers to Tim's question echoes in the room: 'defeat', 'despair', 'frustration', 'helplessness'.

Tim points out that all these emotions can cause us to feel like giving up. He then mimics someone suffering from depression. He slumps forward towards his laptop, his arms folded over his heart, face down, hiding a frown - demonstrating that 'giving up' has both psychological and physical effects.

Tim asks "Is this feeling of helplessness actually helping?" A quick staccato of "No – No – No - No." Someone adds "It's knocking the person's energy down. It's harmful."

The last question in the middle column is 'Is this thought exaggerated or irrational?' Tim adds "This is a tricky question. So pretend to be a lawyer. How would you pick holes in the logic of the distressing thought if you were in court? How would you say the thought isn't quite right? In what way is the thought exaggerated beyond the truth of the situation?"

Cheryl Ann, who now leads a national charity and has worked with a difficult cancer and side effects of her therapy for years, begins, "You can't say that you don't have the strength to do this, because this is the first time you've done this – there's not been a 'before'."

Tim responds, "Right. This is all new territory and the fact is that you *are* getting through this. You're here; you're alive. Therefore, it's actually not really true. You do have the strength."

Anne is trying to get her life on track after being treated for ovarian cancer with surgery and chemotherapy. "Initially, that may be how you feel—from there you can possibly find the strength. I might find a deeper well to draw from."

Tim replies "Yes! That is a beautiful image of new possibilities. You don't want to freeze the situation into a thought or make it true just because you believe it. These thoughts have a lot of power to shape your ongoing experience. If you look closely, you see that the truth is always shifting and changing, never frozen."

The group is starting to see through the "black or white" thinking implied in "It's no use. I don't have the strength."

Tim outlines the idea of relaxing into the experience of not knowing what's going to happen and reminds the group about becoming comfortable with the unknown. "When we panic in the face of the unknown, we tend to generate a lot of thoughts to create an illusion of knowing what's going to happen. This can cause further distress, especially if we have been conditioned to think about 'worst-case scenarios'. This way of thinking can become what is called the fortune-teller error—predicting one's demise.

"The fact is that we don't really know what's going to happen in the future, and so it is better to learn to relax with that truth. Otherwise, thoughts like "I can't cope" and "It's no use" do not help and actually make you feel worse."

Tim guides the group to the right column, and to step back from the distorted thought and look at the whole situation from rational perspective, creating a 'reframe' that is both wise and kind. He asks "What would a loving grandmother say if you shared the distressing thought 'It's no use. I don't have the strength to get through this.' Is there a way to reframe this way of thinking?"

After a long pause, Cheryl Ann volunteers a reframe, "I *have* to get through this. It's non-negotiable. I'll just have to do it!"

Tim is quick to caution about using that tone of voice with oneself. "That sounds like it puts a lot of pressure on you. That's kind of like the pushy angry parent that says, 'You have to do that.'

"But you could say 'I *will* get through this' or 'I *can* get through this' The specific words that you use are very important, because when you're talking to yourself like that you can feel pressure. Be careful of 'should' and 'have to', right? When you say 'I will' or 'I can' it's much kinder to yourself and therefore more encouraging and effective."

Trudy, a retired flight attendant who struggled with leukemia for years, asks, "Is it OK to acknowledge that this is a difficult time?"

"Oh, for certain." Tim continues "It's very important to be honest about how you feel, even about your level of despair. To begin, own your emotions completely. Feel them, and then look at what you can do."

Trudy follows up. "Oh. So, I don't have to do everything all at once. I don't have to eat the whole elephant today."

Tim smiles and continues on this theme. "No, you don't have to! Most important is to be kind to yourself and to pace yourself. Dr. David Burns, who introduced this technique, used the example of imagining all the meals that you eat in your whole life placed in a football stadium. If you were asked to eat all that food, you'd say, 'Oh my god, I could never eat all that food!' But the truth is that over your lifetime that's how much food you will eat. So when you break up the challenge into little bits, it becomes workable and you don't overwhelm yourself—you can take baby steps."

Cora Lee, a young teacher whose husband is facing a bone marrow transplant for an aggressive form of leukemia, says "I just want to add that you can encourage yourself by saying 'I've done hard things before – I can do another one.'"

Tim remarks that Cora Lee has a different tone of voice in this sugges-tion—like a good friend or a wise coach who gives you encouragement to draw on your inner strength and resilience without minimizing the difficulty in the situation. When you develop that wise and compassion-ate part of yourself, you will find many ways that you can help reframe your thinking to take yourself forward.

Tim finishes, "This is just one way to reframe. There's no one best way." He reads the 'Kind and Rationale Response' from the right column of the table: "Who said that I always have to be strong? Sometimes to cry and fall apart is the best thing to do. Then it seems I can find an inner strength, a higher power."

"By going into suffering you may notice that something comes up from within, as was said earlier. You may find a deeper well to draw from or you may allow yourself to be supported by others. When you stay with the feelings without judging them, you start to find that there is a kind of buoyancy and resilience."

Mindful of Distressing and Automatic Thoughts	Inquiry and Insight	Kind and Rational Response
"It's no use. I don't have the strength to get through this."	• What emotions follow this way of thinking? *Despair, frustration, helplessness* • Is this a helpful or harmful thought? *Harmful* • Is this thought exaggerated or irrational? *Yes*	*Who said that I always have to be strong? Sometimes to cry and fall apart is the best thing to do. Then it seems I can find an inner strength, a higher power.*

CHAPTER 24

Geoff
Trading in his Hockey Stick for a Walking Stick

Geoff Eaton stands 6 foot 5, has a mischievous smile and a twinkle in his eye. At age 22, St. John's Newfoundland was his home. Geoff was studying business full-time in university and running his own marketing company. He also played an intense game of hockey and partied often with his friends.

Almost overnight, Geoff seemed to lose his energy. His buddies blew past him on the ice. He chalked this up to his weight, then 225 pounds. One night, turning to place his drink down at a business reception, he fell over backwards and woke up staring at the ceiling. Intuitively he knew his life was about to change dramatically.

The doctors found Geoff had acute myeloid leukemia (AML), a rare and very serious blood cancer. The cancer cells were crowding out the normal blood cells, putting him at risk for severe infections, bleeding, and sapping his life energy. Geoff was given six hours to leave the hospital to prepare for a prolonged hospital admission. Facing six hours that could be his last out in the world, he went to his apartment to get music, gym pants, and his pillow. Twice he went to Signal Hill, the local mountain, overlooking his coastal city. From these heights, a fierce determination was arising. Geoff wanted to do everything possible to watch these sunsets and to drive his motorcycle till age 95. He choked up at the thought of not having an opportunity to breathe life into his dreams. He asked himself over and over what he needed to do to stay alive.

Back in his apartment his roommate cornered him, demanding to know why Geoff looked so upset. Geoff knew the one-word answer to his friend's question but it wouldn't come out. He kept trying to say it. Finally Geoff said clearly "Leukemia, they think it's leukemia."

Geoff thinks that this moment of acknowledging the diagnosis directly was a turning point for him. "It was as if this major weight was taken off my shoulders, the knife taken out of my back. Literally, in that instant, my whole perspective switched and I started to say to my inner self 'Yeah, they think I have leukemia and I can f'ing tackle that!'"

He remembers walking into the hospital elevator for the very first course of chemotherapy. His face was expressionless but the eyes were intense—this was his "game face"—the feeling he got as he walked to the arena before a big hockey game. He would get 'aggressive' with his cancer. He created a virtual play-off hockey series in his head, 'Geoff versus cancer'. Each round of chemotherapy would represent a game in his series. Geoff's family and friends bought into his strategy completely. His Dad brought him his official Mario Lemieux stick; a buddy who works for the St. John's Maple Leafs gave him the official puck; and he wore the same jersey he wore when he captained his high school team. The puck soon became the symbol of his soul energy and stayed with him throughout his hospitalization.

Before every new round of chemotherapy, nurses would set up the IV pole opposite Geoff. Hunched over at the faceoff, stick crossing over the lines of chemotherapy, the puck was dropped. When Geoff played hockey he played to win. He told his physicians that it was his game—not theirs. He was the player and they were the coaches. His family and friends would have to watch from the stands.

Geoff interpreted every symptom as if it arose during a hockey game. If he got a headache from a blood transfusion, he understood that he had taken a hit to the head from his opponent. When his energy levels sagged, he knew he had to get off the ice for a quick rest on the bench. "For me, in some strange way, I felt when I was having pain and discomfort that I was really 'playing hard', competing if you will, and I took comfort from that. It was part of the game."

Geoff brought this same fiery intensity to his interactions with the medical team. Whether the person was a physician, nurse, therapist or cleaning person, if anyone tried to talk down to him, he would 'slam them shut.'

"I'm a 'Proactive Patient', which basically means sometimes I'm a big pain in the ass for docs and nurses, but I always qualified that with 'I hopefully, I'll be equally rewarding.' I wanted to know what the drug side-effects might be and specifically when and how long I would take the drugs." As Geoff's reputation grew, his physicians began to send in medical students to learn from this master in self-advocacy.

Geoff reflects back to this time and says "I had this feeling in my gut that I was going to experience some amazing things, both 'good' and 'not so good'. And I felt I wanted to share those experiences and the lessons

I learned as a result. I was eager to talk to anyone who would listen, and that included medical students. I also started an e-mail group the first week I was in hospital to keep friends and family up to date on my progress. To share my story was one of the most significant decisions I made."

Geoff's treatment plan included a bone marrow transplant with marrow from his Dad. This occurred at a major cancer centre 2000 miles from his home, and required high-dose chemotherapy designed primarily to destroy the leukemia in his body. It would also destroy many healthy cells, including his entire immune system. As a result of this intense treatment, Geoff had to spend forty days of harrowing isolation in a psychological desert—a minor infection could be deadly.

With stick and puck in hand, he began days of chemotherapy. One night, weakened to the point of despair, he slumped over on the toilet. To his left hung his chemotherapy medication dripping in from a big brown bag. On his right hung a bag of red blood cells which flowed in smoothly. He began to think about never being able to play hockey again. Suddenly he felt a presence in the room and a tap on his head. A voice from beyond seemed to say, "You are going to have to choose one or the other"—the brown bag of chemotherapy or the red bag of blood. At that moment he resolved to choose the vibrant red blood...to choose life.

Thus began a slow and painful recovery. The days ticked by. Geoff befriended one of the Jamaican nurses on the unit - Rose. She was boisterous, fun, and full of life. He wanted some independence, and Rose understood this. He asked her to teach him how to unhook the lines and feeding tubes because there was a rock concert in town he wanted to attend. Geoff knew he would expose himself to a sea of germs among the thousands of fans, but he reasoned life is meant to be lived and every decision is a balance of risk and benefit. He loved the concert and, as it turns out, he didn't get sick.

His blood counts continued to improve. After two months cooped up in a hospital room, far from his Newfoundland home, Geoff longed for a view of the ocean. When the doctors gave him the green light, he literally took the next flight home. Puck in hand, donning his hockey jersey, he decided to send his winning stick home by car, worried the airline would break it.

A week after Geoff got home, the party came to a crashing stop. At 3:00 AM, fevers, chills, and a bad set of shakes signalled an infection in the IV line in his upper chest. Back into hospital for high dose antibiotics.

Geoff was sick. Deathly sick. Each day the frown on his doctor's face deepened. A second infection. Plummeting blood counts. Geoff wrote his will and planned his funeral. One organ after another began to shut down—and he became agitated and scared. He was spending what little life energy he had thrashing about.

The doctors wanted to put a tube down his throat, put him on life support, to try to paralyze his muscles in a last effort to save his life. But in Geoff's mind he was still skating hard. He couldn't think clearly. He refused to let the doctors get close enough to place the tube down his throat. He began to lash out at them. His father and brother were pleading with him to let them do it, each holding down a shoulder—a father's nightmare, fighting against a dying son.

The tube went in but Geoff was still punching out, exhausted but not willing to let go of the hockey game. Geoff's dad yelled at him, "Have you had enough?" With a tube finally down his throat, Geoff scrawled a note: "Not yet."

The medication took effect. It required ten times the normal dosage to put down this raging elephant. Geoff was suspended in a deep sleep, barely holding on to life. The next 48 hours were agony for his family. Each hour the update was worse than the one before.

His father arrived at 7:00 AM to disastrous news. Geoff's lungs had begun to bleed. Two respiratory therapists focused on his every breath, suctioning out the pink froth. The team was working wildly around him. Geoff was dying. The chance of recovery was less than one percent.

Meanwhile, Geoff was dreaming he was an infantryman at war, separated from his fellow soldiers, staggering through the deep brush. If only he could find the troops. He stood up in an opening to get a better view of the facing hill. Suddenly enemy fighters jumped up and stitched him with machine gun fire in the chest. He was bleeding into his lungs.

Hour after hour Geoff dangled limp on the brink of death. Nightfall. Darkness everywhere. Waiting. Praying.

Clutched in the palm of Geoff's hand was his hockey puck. Holding. Holding. Even when the nurses adjusted the IVs, they knew not to disturb the puck in his hand. The physiotherapists turned him and stretched him out without displacing his puck. Everyone knew that Geoff wanted to keep playing in this series.

Suddenly someone asked "Where is Geoff's hockey stick?" Someone rushed home to bring it in.

Slowly the numbers on the monitors began to climb upwards, step by step, flashing hope and possibility.

Geoff opened his eyes three weeks later. His family was at his bedside holding their collective breath. He wanted to give his mother a hug, but he was too weak to even lift his arms. They wanted to know if he'd seen the light—gone to the other side and back. Geoff couldn't answer.

Three weeks going through the dark night of the soul had devastated his mental abilities. He had no idea where he was, and he had absolutely no memory of what had happened. He could hardly talk. He started with the basics... 'Where am I? What happened?' He asked those questions repeatedly for days until the answers were firmly planted in his head.

Geoff was terrified of sleeping because he thought that if he fell asleep he'd never wake up again. He was suffering from what doctors call 'ICU psychosis'. It was a restless time of dark thoughts and fear of death.

His mother was the first to see the predicament. She understood that if he didn't sleep, he wouldn't recover. No degree of coddling could settle his fear. Finally, she snapped "If you want to get home, you're going to have to let yourself sleep." Jaw clenched, she walked briskly out of the room.

Geoff looked over at the nurse. He scrawled on the pad, "What do I have to do to get out of this place?" The nurse pointed to the monitor measuring the oxygen in his bloodstream. "You have to get your oxygen saturation greater than 90 percent without the oxygen mask." He squeezed his puck hard once, and then melted into his bed for deep sleep. A few days later he was discharged from intensive care to the medical ward, stable but very weak.

Geoff ran a hand up his abdomen and chest. His muscles had dissolved. His mother had to brush his teeth for him and nurses turned him in bed to wash his backside.

Even though Geoff was mentally and physically exhausted, he couldn't take being in the hospital any longer. He looked at his Mom and said, "I need to go home." The doctors refused, explaining that Geoff would be 100 percent dependent on his family for everything. But the family was ready for the responsibility. On the way home from the hospital, they drove him up to Signal Hill on what was a beautiful sunny August afternoon.

At home, Geoff was so weak he couldn't give his brother a high-five or shake his Dad's hand, never mind get to the bathroom. This was a significant issue for Geoff because the chemotherapy had literally removed the lining of his gut, leaving a problem of unpredictable diarrhea. Thankfully, his great sense of humour was always present. For example, not fully knowing what would happen if he had to pass gas, he would joke with his Dad and say "Let's roll the dice!"

Geoff used his hospital bed for the first stages of his strength training. He tried to raise himself up by pulling on the rails. He did these pull-ups every day and eventually was strong enough to hold himself in the sitting position...next would be getting back on his feet.

Just two and a half weeks after leaving hospital, Geoff made a momentous five-step journey from his hospital bed to his couch. It was a moment of incredible triumph for him. Sitting down, though, Geoff found himself literally swallowed by the couch. He was trapped with no strength to keep himself upright or get back on his feet and make his way back to bed without help.

But Geoff was determined and worked hard. A mere seven months after his first steps, he was back at work. He created a national organization, initially known as RealTime Cancer and now called Young Adults Cancer Canada.

He decided to mark the first anniversary of his first steps to the couch by climbing Signal Hill. He invited 170 of his friends, family, and email buddies to join him in the first Young Adults Cancer Climb. Now this climb is an annual event in many cities.

It is a long walk to the top of Signal Hill. But Geoff was walking up a mental mountain as well. He was taking his healing journey very seriously.

Geoff began to watch his body more closely. He found exercise was crucial to his recovery but noticed that he couldn't attack life at a breakneck pace. He needed nine hours of sleep to stay sharp mentally. He learned to slow down, take time off, and pace himself. He admits this is a work in progress.

An internal transformation was occurring at this time. He no longer viewed his cancer as an enemy. "I didn't hate it anymore. I didn't want it dead—just gone. Cancer is my friend, not a friend I want forever, but it has taught me so many valuable lessons and helped me develop a perspective I would not trade for anything in the world. I began to look at my life more as a journey. I would just take this one step at a time." Geoff had traded in his hockey stick for a walking stick.

Geoff was told that if he could make it to the two-year anniversary date of his bone marrow transplant, he would likely be cured of his leukemia—and if he didn't, his chances were essentially nil.

On the cusp of Geoff's two-year anniversary, however, his blood counts began to plummet. His leukemia had recurred. Even though this news was devastating, Geoff understood it simply as another bump on the road of life.

But this time, there was no more gritting his teeth. Geoff's game face had softened and a calm settled in his eyes. His friends thought he was giving up. They thought he had forfeited the hockey game. But Geoff was simply in a different frame of mind. The previous outward intensity was now focused deep within his soul.

A nursing shortage at the hospital where he received his first bone marrow transplant was creating delays in re-treatment there which was his first option. A bureaucrat in his home province said there had to be a six-week review before Geoff would be considered for a transplant at another center, delaying his second option. The message from the bureaucrats was "Stay on your chemotherapy and wait to see what happens".

Geoff was drawing on his deep will to live in his dealings with the medical system and his determination led him to a third option. He found out that Ottawa offered the same transplant chemotherapy, on an outpatient basis, that he would receive going back to the original hospital. In Ottawa, Geoff could stay in an apartment beside the hospital, ready to rush back if he ever spiked a fever or felt unwell.

He jumped at the chance and went to Ottawa. After the second transplant, he never needed to be readmitted. His leukemia had disappeared for the time being.

Geoff won't pretend that he had no fear of recurrence, but his psychological and spiritual perspective continued to blossom. He sought the help of a counsellor and a few alternative practitioners to help him heal his body and his psyche. After the second transplant, his osteopath, an insightful and wise healer, asked him a life-altering question: "What didn't you learn about yourself during your first remission?"

Geoff had to admit that he had always pushed down his emotions. He considered himself almost like a politician at times, saying what others wanted to hear. He also realized he was angry at being debilitated again and decided to let it out for the first time. "This is bullshit. I don't know how I'm feeling. All I know is I have to drag myself out of bed every day."

"I learned it was okay to be afraid and cry. It's okay to be mad and upset. But for me it's not okay to let myself stay in those places. There is a time and place, but it's not forever."

Geoff decided to buy a motorcycle as part of his recovery—to experience the wind, open spaces, and a rush of joy. He was back hanging with his friends. He had time now to share some laughs with his friend's younger sister, Karen. His friend cautioned him not to get involved with her.

Geoff jokes, "But I had already broken into the fortress to win the princess." Before they knew it, Karen's arms were wrapped around Geoff as they took long rides on his motorcycle. A love affair. Marriage. Lots of learning, listening, and really loving deeply.

How does Geoff feel about having a life-threatening illness and being in a long-term relationship? Does he wish the cancer had never occurred?

Geoff is philosophical in his reply. "I honestly believe that all of our experiences have purpose, nothing is random, and everything has meaning. I believe there's this huge force, I call it the universe, and it connects all of us. While we are here, we can act from one of two main places, love or fear. I like what I experience and what happens in the world around me when I'm coming from the place of love. So I've made the effort to do that. Sometimes I slip, other times I'm golden. It's all part of being human, really."

Four years after his second transplant there was no sign of cancer recurrence. Geoff was a walking miracle. But he was deeply disappointed he couldn't have his own children because his physicians had forgotten to recommend sperm banking before the first chemotherapy. He continued having sperm tests after his second transplant, but always with the same result—no sperm.

Then, one day, he dropped off his little plastic cup and called in to chat with his fertility nurse who told him he had 0.2 million sperm, with motility of 10 percent. "I was jacked! Holy shit, how did that happen? This is still a super low count; but it's a number other than zero and while the boys are barely dancing, they're dancing!

"That fall, my wife and I got in to see a fertility doc to begin talking about our options for starting a family. We had a great chat, but the doc reassured us that my sperm count is like we're using birth control; there was no way we'd have children naturally. What the doc didn't know was that, over the course of the last four years, I had begun to love it when the odds were so strongly stacked against me."

And then came this posting on Geoff's website to the young adult cancer community: "Yes, just after my last super low sperm test, one of my boys beat the odds in a way I never have before. He heard the start gun and gave'er, albeit against a much smaller group of competitors than normal, but that doesn't take away from the victory at all.

"Today, Karen's belly is the biggest it's ever been, she looks the best she's ever looked to me, and in another month or so we'll welcome our little champ into the family.

"So gents, remember, just because you've been given tough news about fertility, just because you've had tests that show your swimmers to be low in numbers, miracles happen!!"

Seven years after his second bone marrow transplant, with no evidence of cancer recurrence, Geoff keeps his hockey puck close by. He returns home every day from his groundbreaking work at Young Adult Cancer Canada—to his wife and two beautiful daughters.

CHAPTER 25

Reframing for the Cancer Hero

Our purpose in life is
to grow in wisdom and in love.
Rachel Naomi Remen

Saturday afternoon. *Every person facing and responding to a cancer diagnosis is unique. While some people are virtually paralyzed by their negative thoughts, many people are very proactive in their approach to the cancer diagnosis. They advocate for themselves and get the best medical care in addition to empowering themselves with specific healing techniques. This approach is laudable for its comprehensive and effective path towards healing the body, mind, and spirit. But if this "I'm going to beat cancer" mentality is taken to the extreme, the proactivity can become an unhealthy obsession.*

To illustrate this to the group, Rob refers to a character called the Cancer Hero, who wants to be just like Lance Armstrong. People who are cancer heroes turn their life into a Tour de France.

Cancer Heroes think that if Lance Armstrong can push himself through the pain of grinding up a mountain for hours, then they should be able to get up at 5:00 AM, go for a 10-mile run, meditate for the next four hours, and spend the rest of the day drinking freshly squeezed vegetable juices. The Cancer Hero might search the Internet late into the night looking for the latest magic cure.

The issue is that Cancer Heroes can become so busy pushing themselves that they fail to appreciate their family and friends and other moments of beauty in their lives. As well, because Cancer Heroes love to fight, the challenge of chemotherapy and other difficult treatments can ignite their fiery determination and they may resolve to push through damaging side effects of therapy with superhuman effort, just as Lance Armstrong drove himself.

This strength and determination is laudable and can carry the Cancer Hero a long way. In the previous chapter, Geoff drew on his soul energy and will to survive to persevere through seemingly unbeatable challenges. Geoff's story also illustrates the natural tendency for most people to want to 'fight' against cancer when first diagnosed. While some may never feel that urge to fight, for Cancer Heroes the fighting response works well and may be helpful throughout their whole cancer journey, or for only part of it.

Wisdom comes in recognizing when to push oneself, and when to take a more moderate approach. It is important to appreciate that each human body has its limits. For example, some types of chemotherapy can cause too much stress on the cellular matrix of certain individuals and, in these instances, the wise approach is to modify the chemotherapy. Unfortunately, Cancer Heroes tend not to pay enough attention to messages from their bodies, and miss out on taking better care of themselves.

Wearing the Cancer Hero mask may work for the first few months, but most people will reach a point in an intense treatment schedule when they physically need a break. Unfortunately, part of the Cancer Hero's psyche shouts "No! I must keep going. I'll do anything to beat this cancer."

Initially, the Cancer Hero may try to suppress the notion that the body has limits, but their wise inner voice won't be silenced, especially if their body is becoming depleted physically and emotionally. Eventually, the voice of the body's wisdom and the Cancer Hero persona will clash in a psychological battle of mythic proportions. The Cancer Hero may have no idea how to untangle this psychological impasse.

Brian Lobel captures the Cancer Hero's dilemma with great humour in a play called *Ball,* based on his own life after being diagnosed with recurrent testicular cancer that required high-dose chemotherapy and a bone marrow transplant. He tells the true story of attending a hospital picnic for cancer survivors. On stage, he dons the cap and tight spandex outfit of a professional cyclist and contemplates his life's purpose.

"I survived my cancer. But what do I win? Lance Armstrong got the Tour de France, speaking gigs, and a ghostwriter. Everyone else gets all this wisdom and depth that only you derive from cancer, but what do I get? If I wasn't going to become a better person because of all of those procedures then I sure as hell better win some kind of competition. Competition! I need to be a hero. A role model. A SURVIVOR! I know that I will probably never be the best role model or ideal survivor—but I will die trying."

Brian picks up a hula hoop. He explains to the audience he's at a hospital picnic and the organizers have just announced "The Stem Cell Transplant Reunion Picnic Hula Hoop Contest", and he's there to win at all costs.

"Eight cute little daughters of stem cell transplant patients versus Brian Lobel, the world's most competitive cancer survivor. It will be a race to the finish, a fight to the death. Winner take all! (The prize was a Coleman folding lawn chair!) The world needed to see who the real cancer-survivor-turned-hula-hoop-champion was... and so, I hula'd. [Brian begins to hula on stage] If it was a title that Lance Armstrong would never hold, then I would hold it, and so I focused, intensely, passionately..."

The competition is stiff, but Brian is outlasting his much younger competitors until, with only three contestants still in the running, he starts to think about his mother and how she's held his hand through the toughest point in the chemotherapy. Then he snaps out of his reminiscence and tells himself, "Focus, Brian!"

He sneers at the two remaining girls. The judges ask the three of them to take a giant step to the right in an attempt to interrupt their concentration. Brian leaps right, focused on his goal. One of the girls loses her hoop. He has only one girl left to beat.

His mind drifts again to all the visitors coming in to see him in the hospital, laughing and listening with love and tenderness. Suddenly, he realizes that life is not a competition. A tear comes to his eye and his hoop drops to the ground. The competition is over, the last little girl wins, but Brian walks away feeling peaceful and happy.

Brian's performance is refreshing in its honesty and humour. He makes an important point in highlighting how inadequate he felt when he compared himself to Lance Armstrong. This is a valuable insight—that there is no way that we can be a hero like anyone other than our own true self. Finding our way through a labyrinth of suffering, fear, and pain, and confronting our own demons is the only way that we can go. In this way, each person is an extraordinary hero in his or her own right.

We've seen Cancer Hero personalities find ways to reframe their thoughts with a peaceful approach. Carol, a very determined French-Canadian woman with breast cancer, had a moment of insight when, in the midst of chemotherapy, she had the rational thought that maybe the treatment was too much for her.

At that moment, her thinking changed from, "I have to do this" to "I don't know if I can." Suddenly a great pressure was released and she felt liberated—she could let go of the demanding voice within. She acknowledged her needs and asked for help. Her nausea medication was adjusted, enabling her to breeze through the rest of that cycle of chemotherapy, and, by the next cycle of treatment, she could eat whatever she wanted.

Kathy told a similar story. The first time she was treated for Hodgkin's lymphoma, she regarded her chemo as an inconvenience. In classic Cancer Hero fashion, she never really considered her own mortality, figuring she'd just do chemo and get on with things.

When Kathy later developed simultaneous recurrent lymphoma and liver failure, she was shaken to the core. There appeared to be no reasonable treatment options, and both diseases directly threatened her life. Like the Cancer Hero pushed beyond his limits, she felt that she was doing absolutely everything possible for herself but was getting nowhere. Positive and healthy reframing was critical for her at this point.

"Being a strong person, I had to learn how to surrender to the possibility that I might die. That possibility was a fact I couldn't deny. So to reframe, I had to go really close to the thought that 'Maybe I won't survive' before I came to be at peace with this."

Kathy was able to relax into the unknown. Instead of trying to control everything, she began to accept and love herself for how she was feeling in each moment. Acknowledging honestly that there were some things beyond her control, she gradually learned to soften even in the face of her worst fears.

By reframing, Kathy shed a whole layer of unnecessary suffering and self-torment. When she let go of trying to control everything, her body was better able to heal. Now, several years later, after reframing her Cancer Hero persona, she is a walking miracle.

CHAPTER 26

Reframing Distressing Thoughts with Kindness and Insight

The essence of practice is always the same.....
we gradually learn to catch the emotional
reaction and drop the story lines.
Pema Chrödrön

Saturday afternoon. *Tim takes the group through a few more examples of common distressing thoughts that those with a cancer diagnosis, and their loved ones, often have, and shows the group how they can be reframed.*

Tim emphasizes there is no one best way to reframe any particular distressing thought. The 'reframes' seen in the right column of the tables are simply examples of how to look at the situation differently - with wisdom and kindness.

Being aware of how our *thoughts* about a situation can be different from the *reality* of the situation is especially important in our relationships. For example, if you think, "My spouse/partner is unsupportive. She/he should be helping me more", your thoughts are framing the situation with your expectations. There may be a lot more that you do not see. Maybe your spouse is actually scared and needs support, not judgment. Maybe your spouse doesn't know what would be helpful and needs practical advice about what to do. Maybe your spouse could be very supportive, but thinks you need space.

Over the years, a number of people attending the retreats have continued to angrily point the finger at the situation and reject the possibility of seeing the world from a different perspective. When they keep thinking 'My spouse is not doing enough to support me', they tend to miss the first important step of acknowledging that their thoughts about their spouse are causing most of their anger. The opportunity to really practice the life-altering skill of reframing is lost.

Learning to reframe takes practice and mindfulness of the distressing thoughts that often pass through our minds. Once we recognize the thoughts we can begin to work with them. The best way to learn this technique is to practice by following through several examples.

Example 1 – "I'll handle this myself"

The situation: This elderly woman is deeply loved by many people in her life. She has given of herself constantly to her family and friends, and rarely, if ever, asked for help from others. When her cancer treatments make her body weak to the point where she can no longer cope on her own, she becomes frustrated and angry at her situation.

Her distressing and automatic thought is "I'm the one that always takes care of others. I can't bear asking for help. I'll handle this myself."

Step 1: Write down the distressing thought. (Left column, facing page)
By acknowledging that these thoughts are just thoughts, and don't define exactly what is happening, she can begin to look at her situation in a different way. In fact she may begin to perceive some of the underlying assumptions that lead to this way of thinking. She may also realize that she's creating frustration by simultaneously thinking 'I'll handle this myself' while actually wishing that someone would help her.

Step 2: Inquiry and Insight (Middle column)
These thoughts are causing her to feel resentment, frustration, anger, helplessness and more. They are not helpful.

"Always" is an exaggeration. "I can't bear asking for help" is irrational. Would she go insane if someone gave her a ride to the cancer centre?

Step 3: Kind and Rationale Response (See the right column)
"It is scary" acknowledges that this is a difficult situation for her. We're not trying to minimize, or simply apply 'positive thoughts' on top of her distress. She can be kind to herself and accept her situation fully, including the fact that her thoughts are distorted based on habitual thinking patterns from the past. From this starting place, she can find a new way of thinking that opens up new possibilities for relating with others.

She could 'reframe' that when she lets others help her, she is actually giving them a precious gift. This change in perspective may be what works for this loving lady.

Mindful of Distressing and Automatic Thoughts	Inquiry and Insight	Kind and Rational Response
I'm the one that always takes care of others. I can't bear asking for help. I'll handle this myself.	• What emotions follow this way of thinking? *Resentment, frustration, and anger* • Is this a helpful or harmful thought? *Harmful* • Is this thought exaggerated or irrational? *Both*	*It is scary but maybe now it is my time to receive and be open to the love and compassion of friends and family. I can consider this a spiritual lesson about the circle of giving and receiving.*

Example 2 – "Cancer is ruining everything"

The situation: A middle-aged couple retired early to spend more time together, biking and walking around the city, and travelling extensively. When his wife is weakened by cancer spread to her bone, the husband is angry about the cancer diagnosis and that their life together is much more sedentary.

His distressing and automatic thought: "I hate this cancer. It's ruining our lives and all the things we do together."

Step 1: Write down the distressing thought (Left column, next page).
By writing down his distressing thought, the husband can see exactly what he's *thinking*, and separate that from the natural level of anger that comes up in this situation. The idea is to identify the extra/unnecessary suffering by seeing the ways that his thinking is adding to his anger.

A key concept in reframing is to see the thoughts about a situation as separate from the situation. Thoughts are only an interpretation, one narrow view of a situation. Thoughts do not define the whole picture. As we have learned before, our thoughts are like the map - not the territory. Because we are fooled, over and over, by believing our thoughts, we forget to look at things with an inquisitive mind. We can end up in a trance of our own making. Then labelling something as good or bad, we end up reacting to the labels and fail to see the complex and ever changing truth underneath.

Step 2: Inquiry and Insight (Middle column)

The emotions that arise from thinking 'the cancer is ruining everything' are anger and frustration, and a feeling of helplessness. He is giving a lot of power to the idea of 'cancer.' It is not helpful to dwell on the physical limitations they are experiencing in their lives.

By paying careful attention to the choice of words, he can identify the exaggeration. 'Hate' and 'ruining' are very strong words. 'Ruining everything and '*all* we do' are both untrue because undoubtedly there are some aspects of their lives that have been maintained – including expressing their love for each other.

Step 3: Kind and Rational Response (Right column)

An honest and wise approach is needed in this very difficult situation. There has been a tremendous change in their lives, and their expectations of what they would do in their retirement have been dashed. Now is the time to bring in that wise elder's voice, which can clearly see what's happening and who cares deeply about this man. (See right column)

Mindful of Distressing and Automatic Thoughts	Inquiry and Insight	Kind and Rational Response
I hate this cancer. It's ruining our lives and all the things we do together.	• What emotions follow this way of thinking? *Anger, fear, and helplessness* • Is this a helpful or harmful thought? *Harmful* • Is this thought exaggerated or irrational? *Exaggerated*	*Anger, rage, and hate only make me feel worse and add to stress for the whole family. With acceptance, I can enjoy the time we do have. We may not be as active, but our time together is very precious.*

Example 3 — 'I have to be the strong one'

The situation: The woman from the previous scenario is going through chemotherapy and can see that her husband is upset. Trying to protect him from further hurt, she doesn't want to burden her husband with her own feelings of worry and sadness.

Her distressing and automatic thought: "I have to be the strong one. I can't let him know how I really feel. If I fall apart, that will make it worse for him."

Unfortunately this type of thinking creates more barriers in their relationships. The wife may feel more alone and unsupported if she acts this way. Her husband may interpret her unwillingness to share her own obvious distress as a sign that she doesn't want him to share his feelings either. Her attempts to "stay positive" leave them both wearing the happy mask for each other and hiding their true emotions.

Step 1: Write down the distressing thought (Left column, next page)
By writing it down, she is taking the first necessary step of seeing the thought as a thought — and not the totality of the truth. Thoughts about how 'I have to be' or 'should' behave or what another person 'should' or 'shouldn't' do within a relationship are based on conjecture and expectations, and are distortions that cause further grief and anger. In a relationship we need to check our assumptions with the other person by asking them directly what they want and need.

Step 2: Inquiry and Insight (Middle column, next page)
The thought 'I have to be the strong one' is not helpful in that it causes her to feel more emotional distance from her husband. 'Have to be' and 'can't' are clues to exaggerated and distorted thinking.

If this woman thought about the situation and her thinking more closely she may be able to see logical flaws in her view. For instance, if she continues to think and act in this way, her husband will continue to feel excluded from her inner life. If she would just be honest and open with her own natural emotions, he could comfort her as he has done in past. Their roles could switch back and forth as need be; they could be drawn closer together on their journey.

She is also making an assumption that her falling apart will make him feel worse.

Step 3: Kind and Rational Response (Right column)
This woman has gained insight from her answers in the middle column.
She can now see a way to reframe the thought she had in the first place
that will be better for her and her husband.

Mindful of Distressing and Automatic Thoughts	Inquiry and Insight	Kind and Rational Response
I have to be the strong one. Can't let him know how I really feel. *If I fall apart, that will make it worse for him.*	• What emotions follow this way of thinking? *Emotional distance with her husband* • Is this a helpful or harmful thought? *Harmful* • Is this thought exaggerated or irrational? *False assumptions*	*It's best to be honest with each other about our feelings. Creates more intimacy, and is truly supportive. If I fall apart how do I know it will make him feel worse? Maybe consoling me will make him feel better.*

Another Way to Look at the Three-column Technique

The three column technique can help you to look at your own thoughts,
learn which thoughts cause further suffering, and then train yourself
in a new way of thinking. Each column draws on a different aspect of
your mind. According to transactional analysis, the 'child' ego state (left
column) tends to think in ways that are irrational or inaccurate; the
'adult' ego state (middle column) can step back with insight and logic
to examine a thought; and, finally, the 'parent' ego state (right column) is
capable of reframing the thought in a way that is both kind and helpful.
The important thing is to observe the conversations that you have with
yourself and identify these different roles, remembering that you can reframe your thoughts.

Seeing these three columns as the three ego states of child, adult, and
parent, puts a human face on these internal dynamics. We can be more
understanding when we know it is the 'child' part of our self who thinks

in distorted ways. Then, when we can identify and separate out the logical adult, it becomes very clear that some of our thoughts are distorted. Finally, we can learn to re-parent ourselves with loving kindness as we create a nurturing parent voice that encourages and guides us with a reframe that is both true and helpful.

The Power of Practice

Undoing old habits and developing new approaches takes time. It often helps if you do something concrete, like actually using the three-column table and writing down your thoughts, insights and reframes. By using the table many times, over a period of weeks or months, you realize that distorted thoughts arise in your mind more frequently than you might have noticed. If you observe a repetitive distressing thought, this is usually a clue to underlying unresolved issues and there's more work to do. Enlisting the help of a trained professional like a psychologist or a counsellor may also be helpful in the process.

As you practice reframing together with mindfulness and meditation, the natural intelligence within your mind begins to make connections between certain ways of thinking and certain painful emotions. As you develop awareness of this 'cause and effect' relationship between distorted thinking and feelings of hopelessness, depression or anger that follow, you gradually develop the insight and skill to transform your own distortions. As you delve further and further into your deepest core beliefs, and begin to see that much of your perception of the world is held in your thinking, you can let go of many assumptions, and be released into a world of possibility and spaciousness.

Remember to be kind to yourself. Gentleness and persistence are both essential for bringing about a change in your thoughts and attitudes – and in redirecting you to the natural capacity for peace and simple joy that are always there in your mind and heart.

CHAPTER 27

Jackie
Working Towards Forgiving Myself

Jackie is a bubbly and strong-willed 45-year-old woman immersed in the fullness of life. The mother of five children, ages nine to twenty-one, she has worked as a psychology assistant, is highly competent and organized, and is used to "taking care of the world." In the small group with six other retreat participants, however, she courageously exposed the private, inner nightmare of her most distressing thoughts, and how hard she can be on herself.

"Four years ago when I first developed breast cancer, I was paralyzed by the diagnosis. After treatment, I went for more tests, including a bone scan. There was one little spot on my shoulder, but the radiologist said it was highly unlikely to be cancerous and, essentially, my family doctor said 'You're fine.' So I didn't ask to see the results. I was just like a bunny in the headlights.

"Then two years later I got a sore shoulder. I went to have another bone scan and, lo and behold, the spot was bigger and it was cancer.

"Now I feel so guilty. I feel guilty that I was so paralyzed by my fear that I didn't take very good care of myself. If I had seen that bone scan result, even if they had said it was highly unlikely, I would have said 'Sorry, stick a needle in there. I can't sleep until I know.' If they had found out it was cancer, I think they would have given me a more aggressive chemo, and I might still be in remission. I feel so guilty because I'm afraid that this disease is going to take me away from my kids.

"Whenever I think about this, I say to myself 'You stupid idiot! You're always being so bloody emotional, you became so paralyzed by fear, and you didn't do anything about it. You didn't take care of yourself.' Jackie stopped to reflect. "I know I shouldn't say that to myself, but I do."

She looked around her small group, exasperated. Her hair was just starting to grow back after her fourth line of chemotherapy. She was having difficulty seeing how to reframe her distressing thoughts.

In Jackie's case, the facts are she didn't ask to see the results of her first bone scan. She doesn't know if the delay in discovering the spread of cancer will shorten her life. (Medically speaking, it probably made no difference at all).

Jackie read out her automatic and distressing thought from the left column on her page: "You stupid idiot! You are always being so bloody emotional. You became so paralyzed by fear and you didn't do anything about it. You didn't take care of yourself. And now this disease is going to take you away from your kids." Her voice was unsteady, caught between anger with herself and a deep sense of sadness.

Jackie sat back and had a good look at the middle column titled "Inquiry and Insight" to think about how her distressing thought was affecting her. She admitted that "When I think 'I'm a stupid idiot!' I become fearful and depressed. I feel so guilty and I have a great deal of difficulty living today when I say those things to myself."

Then Jackie began to examine to what degree her distressing thought was actually true. She acknowledged right away that the "stupid idiot" part is an exaggeration, irrational, not true, and a label she slaps on herself when she lapses into a juvenile form of thinking. Likewise, she could see the line, "You are always being so bloody emotional" is an unjustified judgment and an overgeneralization, spoken like the harsh voice of her father that she has been repeating to herself for years. Beginning to see through this misconception, she realized it did not really pertain to her and added "The 'always' makes the statement irrational and untrue because, most of the time I am clear-headed and rational. I do have my moments, but that's just it, they are moments, not 'always' or 'all the time.'"

The group challenged her to question the statements "You didn't do anything about it." and "You didn't take care of yourself." She told the group she had done many things to take care of herself, but she was feeling guilty and angry with herself because she had followed her doctor's recommendation rather than taking the initiative to follow up on one early test result.

One of the group members pushed her on this point. "Let me get this straight. Are you expecting that you, in your state of shock and early naiveté about cancer, should have known more than your doctor who has studied and worked with cancer for years?"

Jackie reluctantly admitted that this was asking a lot of herself. But, clearly, she was still struggling with being stuck in guilt and judgment of herself.

In the right column, titled "A Kind and Rational Reframe", Jackie tried to develop a creative and helpful alternative to the distressing thought. She tried talking to herself as if she were a wise grandmother or her closest friend who might say "You're not a stupid idiot. You're a highly intelligent woman who is very effective at doing many different things. You may think that you made a mistake when you didn't ask for the test results. You might have, you might not have. Even if you did, we're all human and we all make mistakes."

However, Jackie quickly admitted that this was hard to do because she tends to be very hard on herself, seldom offering herself kind words of reassurance or rational explanations that can help her to feel better.

Jackie drew a deep breath and read her reframe to the group from the right column. "Knowing the cancer had metastasized may have resulted in a longer remission. But it was very normal to be paralyzed with fear at that time."

After a heavy pause and a deep sigh, Jackie shook her head and said "I know I wrote those words but they don't make me feel any better."

Tim was facilitating her small group and asked Jackie to read her reframe again slowly, with kindness, and to let the words sink in. After a pause and a deep exasperated sigh, Jackie suddenly blurted out "I'm probably going to die and my kids aren't going to have a mother. That's going to be so hard for them. I know I'm human… but I want to be better than that… for them." At first wide-eyed and feisty, she then looked down, her eyes filled up, and her lip quivered.

For a long moment, the whole group sat in silence, holding the painful truth of what she was saying. The group also became aware of an oddly humorous quality of her grandly heroic but deeply ironic intention "I know I'm human… but I want to be better than that".

When Jackie spoke again, she seemed to be having a dialogue with herself. The group listened patiently as she gradually worked out the confused framework of logical inconsistencies and knots of emotional pain.

Her voice was calm. "I know it was too much to expect of me at that time. I was so terrified. And I didn't have any experience with cancer. I had never seen anyone or known anyone with cancer. So I don't think I knew to ask for the results at that time. But it sucks so badly. It's such a big consequence for not knowing and being human – for just being normal and fearful.

"But this is what I do…I judge myself all the time. When I was pregnant with my first child and decided not to marry the father, I was becoming almost obsessive in my criticism of myself. But eventually I turned it around and said, 'Hang on. I'm going to be a mom. How am I going to treat this little baby?' I started talking to myself as if I were my child. I told myself 'You're not perfect. Human beings make mistakes and things happen. And everything is going to be okay.' That's the part that I really want to believe now…that I did the best I could, and my kids will be okay." Jackie was not asking for a miracle. She simply wanted her children to thrive regardless of her outcome.

Wendy, also with a breast cancer diagnosis and children of her own, put a hand on Jackie's shoulder and asked her to read her reframe one more time, as if she was saying it to one of her children. In a much softened and more compassionate voice, Jackie read "Knowing the cancer had metastasized may have resulted in a longer remission. But it was very normal to be paralyzed with fear at that time."

This time she believed herself and the sense of her forgiveness was palpable.

CHAPTER 28

Reframing
"You're supposed to stay positive"
A Discussion

There is nothing either good nor bad
but thinking makes it so.
William Shakespeare

Saturday afternoon. *At the beginning of a large group discussion, Tim shares his views about the possible pitfalls of 'positive thinking' as a way to open up discussion.*

"Being positive" has its place on the cancer journey. People who maintain a happy demeanour and envision a hopeful future usually use active coping strategies like negotiating for the best care from the medical system. They take better care of their bodies and nurture their relationships with others. Feeling happy boosts immune system function and helps unleash the innate healing potential in their bodies. With a more positive attitude, they can see through difficult scenarios more easily, taking appropriate action when necessary.

Catch phrases like "the power of positive thinking" or the importance of "the mind-body connection" appear frequently and most people with a cancer diagnosis don't want to see their family and friends suffer. As a result, it is common to don the happy mask. But the pressure, from oneself or others, to always be positive can be exhausting, especially given the reality of the situation.

Contemplating mortality, mourning the loss of one's previous life, dealing with physical side effects of cancer and its treatment, worrying about the future and the effect of a diagnosis on family members – can all weigh heavily. Given that it's both normal and expected to experience a wide range of emotions that accompany a cancer diagnosis, our true face can show anger or fear, or tear up in sadness.

If you believe that you should remain positive even when you're feeling awful, you'll probably feel like you are wrestling with yourself. If you try desperately to hold up the happy mask, straining with all your might to fulfill the expectations of yourself and others, you will create more turmoil. By learning to reframe the thought "I have to stay positive all the time", you can learn to be more genuine, and look at the whole situation with wisdom and kindness.

Tim shares the following as a sample thought: "They say you're supposed to stay positive, but I feel awful, angry, helpless, and filled with despair. I'm afraid that I'm making this worse." He then asks if anyone can identify with this thought. At least half the participants raise their hands.

Mindful of Distressing and Automatic Thoughts	Inquiry and Insight	Kind and Rational Response
"They say you're supposed to stay positive, but I feel awful, angry, helpless, and filled with despair. I'm afraid that I'm making this worse."	• What emotions follow this way of thinking? • Is this a helpful or harmful thought? • Is this thought exaggerated or irrational?	

Tim starts by trying to put them at ease. "This is a complex issue. There may be lots of truth incorporated in this thought because the alternative, openly and publicly wallowing in misery, might make things worse. At the same time, just putting on a happy mask, denying your underlying emotions, doesn't seem wise either.

"We want to start with acknowledging the truth—in this situation you're feeling awful. So let's just take it one step at a time. The first question in the middle column is: What emotions come up when you're thinking 'I feel awful and I'm making this worse'?"

Someone quickly volunteers "Guilt." There's a barrage of other suggestions: "Despair", "Helplessness", "Anger," "Blame and shame". The group is fired up.

Tim throws out another distressing thought: "I'm the cause of my own problems." People are leaning forward in their chairs and comments are arriving on top of each other: "I'm supposed to be happy so I can't even ask for help." and "Nobody wants to be around me because I'm so grumpy."

It's clear that similar internal conversations have been held inside the participants' minds for too long. People are rapidly acknowledging how they've been feeling and are reliving their frustrations. The group is going into a mini frenzy.

Tim jumps in. "Let's move on so you don't get caught in a downward spiral of distressing thoughts. If you allow yourself to get caught in this thinking, your body loses energy." People nod their heads in agreement.

Tim asks, "So is it harmful or helpful to think this way?"

A thin elderly lady with breast cancer starts off but she wants to comment on the underlying issue. Her view of the world has been shaped by years of experience, and she wants to challenge the premise that trying to be positive all the time is beneficial. "I think you need to feel those negative emotions. If not, you're in a type of denial. And we all go through these emotions. Eventually you will say, 'I've got to do something about this. I can't keep on feeling sorry for myself.' But first, you naturally go through the 'Why me?' phase."

Tim emphasizes that difficult feelings are to be expected. "It's normal and natural to go through these emotions. Sometimes you're even going to hold onto them for a period of time. If you're really down, you may decide to see someone to get help. But learning to observe your thoughts with mindfulness is the first step because then you can ask yourself, 'Is it helpful to think this way?'

"With insight, you can possibly see the thought itself as the cause of your inner conflict and pain. It isn't helpful to be ruminating 'I feel awful but I should be positive' over and over again. And so next comes the question: 'How can I reframe this?' How can I see life from a bigger perspective that will allow me to feel better?"

Carol, a young woman recovering from chemotherapy, wants to follow up on the comment about acknowledging negative emotions. "I call it letting the poison out. I read a lot of books about the mind-body connection and I do believe in it, but there are times when you just don't feel right—you know, you don't feel good. But if you let these emotions out, it's positive because you're not letting them stress you out any more.

You're releasing the bad mood. The alternative is to wallow in the bad mood until it becomes ridiculous. Eventually you will have had enough of it. It's like eating too much chocolate."

A young woman, who's supporting her husband on the weekend, points out the consequences of suppressing our emotions: "When I hold back what I'm really feeling, I actually crash even harder when I do crash."

Tim nods and then uses his hands (one pushing up and the other pushing down) to illustrate the tension of suppressing ones emotions. He goes on to explain another idea. "There's a reason for those emotions. They are flowing through us. There's grief. There's loss. We need to honour them, and let them flow. And then we can feel better. There is a natural flow to the process of our emotions, but when our thinking is distorted, we can get stuck."

Tim points out that if we resist our deep sadness for a long time, it will always chase after us. But if we embrace it, the emotion will flow through us. Quoting one of the participants at the retreat "What you resist persists, and what you can embrace transforms."

Kathy, a 47-year-old executive, speaks next. She has been treated for cancer twice and now works with the ongoing problems of liver failure. She points up at the thought in the left column and says "Two of the most harmful words for me are 'supposed to.'" She then recounts her experience with cancer the first time. "All my neighbours marvelled at how I got through cancer. They said, 'You're so up, it's so wonderful.' Then another person in the neighbourhood went through cancer treatment and was in despair. My friends said, 'Kathy, you have to talk to her because she's not handling it'. But I said 'she is handling it; she's just handling it the way she needs to handle it.'"

Kathy continues "You hear that 'supposed to' all the time. But what's right for one person is not necessarily best for the next. All I have to do is know who I am. I'll react the way I'm going to react." Kathy has no interest in trying to deceive anyone—especially herself.

Patty has lived a full life, from growing beyond a dysfunctional family to deciding to marry a loving man who has end-stage prostate cancer. Patty looks over at Kathy. "I agree. I read about a woman who lets herself grieve, and fall into it. Every day she gives herself 15 minutes to really feel all her pain. At the end of 15 minutes, if that doesn't do it for her, she gives herself another 15 minutes. But then she says 'Enough is enough!' and brings herself out of it."

Patty continues, "For me, after I've given myself enough time to grieve, I decide to go for a walk, or get a change of scenery, or phone someone who can listen to me. And this works for me. So I let myself feel awful and honour my grief, and then I take steps to feel better, but only after I feel the pain. Because, if you ignore the pain, then you're not doing yourself a favour. In fact, you're trivializing the situation, which is more harmful than grieving it."

Tim steps forward to clarify an important point. "We need to learn to separate thinking and feeling. The feelings are going to be there and they're going to go up and down. But when we put a label on the emotion and judge ourselves as bad for having that emotion, we're creating an extra level of suffering."

He asks the group: "Is there any distortion in these thoughts: 'They say you're supposed to stay positive, but I feel awful, angry, and helpless and filled with despair. I'm afraid that I'm making this worse'?"

Christine responds, "'*They* say you're supposed to...' Who says? Who is 'they'? We don't have to choose to act a certain way just because society thinks we should."

Tim encourages this type of rational thinking "Right. I want those lawyer types to cross examine this first sentence. What is the logical flaw in 'People say you have to stay positive'?"

Stuart, who happens to be a lawyer, answers directly. "We over generalize when we say the word 'should'. Each person has their own way of handling a situation. You can't expect everyone to react the same way. That would be unrealistic."

Someone else adds "My red flag goes up whenever there is a 'should' in a sentence. Or 'supposed to' or 'always' or 'have to'. I'm uncomfortable with that black-and-white thinking."

Tim asks "So how do we reframe this way of thinking? How do we work with this real life scenario? What would you say to that person who is feeling awful and guilty about not being positive? Can they look at the scenario in a bigger way?"

Christine, who spent years debilitated from her cancer before making an amazing recovery, starts the reframing process. "It's tough to be positive all the time. I just can't be positive 100 percent of the day. And there's no data that feeling awful is necessarily making me worse."

Cheryl Ann, who worked long hard hours to move up the corporate ladder before she developed leukemia, comments, "Sometimes I think back to before my diagnosis when I was working long hours. I would have days when I was off emotionally for no reason at all. So I would say in this situation 'This is just an off day for me. Maybe my off days aren't related to cancer at all.'"

Tim echoes Cheryl Ann's comment. "Yeah, it's normal to have an off day. That's human. Well done."

Tim then refers to the image of a hurricane over the ocean as a metaphor of the emotional turmoil of being given a cancer diagnosis? At the level of the surface of the water, there's a lot of psychological turbulence. But 40 feet down in the water, there appears to be great peace. So when you have emotional turmoil in your life, you can realize the waves of distress are only on the surface, while underneath is a deep resource of stillness and wisdom. Try looking at your distress from this perspective and be kind to yourself. Rather than feeling guilty or being hard on yourself, which only compounds the problem, this is the time for kindness and love and slowing down. Then you can say, 'I'll get through these waves of distress. I need to take care of myself.'

"What we say in the psychology of meditation is that everything is workable. There is nothing that isn't workable. We can actually work with the energy as it is. When we tell ourselves that we can't, then we get into trouble.

"Instead you can tell yourself: 'I don't have to be a certain way. I don't have to be perfect. I don't have to always feel good. There's no 'should'. Instead I honour what is.'"

Cheryl Ann has just had an "aha!" moment. "Something here really resonated for me. Usually, when I am feeling negative, I try to quickly shut that feeling away and say, 'I don't want to feel this way.' Nobody wants to see those negative things, right? But now I see I can actually hold onto those emotions. I can say to myself, 'At this moment in time, that is what I'm feeling. I'm going through it.' Later I can ask 'What am I going to do?' But, I can start by just deciding to hold the emotions in a bigger space."

Tim adds "That's what meditation does. You look at things. You let a thought or an emotion arise. You look at it, feel it, and let it go. We call that 'touch and go'. Don't make a storyline about it; don't make logic around it or place judgement on it. Just see it, feel it, and let it go. This way, things move through you and your natural growth takes place. If you simply and gently honour what is, then natural healing occurs."

Mindful of Distressing and Automatic Thoughts	Inquiry and Insight	Kind and Rational Response
"They say you're supposed to stay positive, but I feel awful, angry, helpless, and filled with despair. I'm afraid that I'm making this worse."	• What emotions follow this way of thinking? *Guilt, frustration…* • Is this a helpful or harmful thought? *Harmful* • Is this thought exaggerated or irrational? *Exaggerated*	*It's natural to have strong and negative feelings. I am learning to comfort myself and ask for reassurance from others. I can work with my state of mind and that helps.*

CHAPTER 29

Karen
All for the Children

As she approached her fortieth birthday, Karen's life was going very well. She worked part time as a physician, timing her shifts with her husband so one of them would always be home with their young children. Karen clearly recalls a strong premonition that this would all change. She had told her mother, the summer before, that things were too perfect. She felt that something was going to happen, there would be a bump in the road, and she prayed that it wouldn't happen to one of her children. But 'it' happened to her – she was diagnosed with breast cancer.

Now, eighteen months after her diagnosis, at the end of the "thought reframing" discussion, Karen stands before the group, curly hair growing in, her blue eyes kind and intelligent. But her usual strong and confident stance begins to shake. "The only thought that I can't really deal with is worrying about my children being left without me. They're so small – they're four and seven. Any of the other fears that I had when I was first diagnosed I was able to work through."

Her voice trembles as she continues: "How can I come to terms with the thought of my children being motherless at such a young age? As a parent, I've done everything to try to be there for my kids in little ways. To contemplate not being there in such a huge way brings a tremendous amount of guilt." She cries unabashedly, demonstrating her deep love and the strength of her maternal bond.

Most of Karen's story is familiar to the group. She discovered her cancer when she felt lumps under her armpit and a mass in her breast. "I'm a doctor! I just freaked out because I knew immediately that it was bad. I dissolved in tears and couldn't spit out the words to verbalize to my husband what I'd discovered. I remember the look on his face was like 'what's going on?'

"The kids were always around so I could only fall apart according to their schedules and when time allowed. I remember pulling myself together and speaking with the surgeon very rationally on the phone. For one appointment, I had my three-year-old daughter with me in his office and had to be very matter-of-fact and normal in front of her."

Karen had her breast and armpit lymph nodes removed, underwent six months of aggressive chemotherapy, five weeks of radiation treatments, and started a five-year course of hormone treatment—all with the intent of curing her breast cancer.

At first, the thought of dying was very difficult and really never left her mind. Karen found herself looking at all the other mothers and children when she attended the Mother's Day Tea at her daughter's preschool. She'd wonder if there would be a time when she wouldn't be able to attend events like her son's Christmas concert. It was hard for her to reign in the melodrama going on in her head about what might be in her children's future.

It was also difficult to decide what to tell her young children about the cancer. For Karen's three year old daughter, the decision was relatively easy. "We told her I had a 'boo boo.' And when my hair started falling out, she would pull on her own hair and say, 'My hair's pretty glued on.' She was matter of fact. In the beginning, she cried a few times when I didn't have my scarf or wig on and she would say, 'Mommy, put your wig on,' but she even got used to that."

Telling her six-year-old son was trickier, especially because he had heard that his Grandpa Hank had died of cancer. At first Karen tried to protect her son from the word "cancer" by saying that she had a "lump" removed. Then Karen's sister suggested it might be best if Karen were the one to tell him because he might hear about her "cancer" from someone at school. Karen agreed.

"That way I could control the message. And it kind of came up naturally one day. My son asked 'Is that lump ever going to come back?' and I told him the lump was a kind of cancer but I was getting treatment for it. He asked 'Is it the dying kind?' He was really into weather at that time, so I said 'Cancer is kind of like the wind. There is the force 10 wind where the roof gets ripped off and then there's the force 0-1 wind where the flag is completely flat. Grandpa Hank had a 10 that was a really bad one and Mommy's got something like a 5—the flag is not completely limp, but it's not a 10 either. That's why I'm getting the strong medicine—to make sure that it doesn't become a 10.

"I felt I was being honest with him without being scary. I don't think you want to leave a kid with anxiety and uncertainty. I know he felt free to bring it up again because he'd say, 'I heard something on the radio about breast cancer. That's the kind you have. They're researching new treatments.' It was completely acceptable to him. But he was sad about my hair loss."

Having cancer allowed Karen's kids to have more time with her. It wasn't all high quality time, but she was around day and night. She stopped working as a doctor, volunteering in the classroom more often. She was there for every bedtime, which was not typical of her life before cancer.

Early on in her journey, Karen wondered if she should begin to create an album or videotape collection for her children in case she died. "My first reaction was to make videotapes for the kids and write extended long letters for them, so they could remember what I was like and all of that. I think that's what tortures a lot of children who lose a parent—the parent becomes a ghost, an outline with nothing filled in. But as the year went on, I thought 'Why do I want to pour energy into something that is predicated on a bad outcome?' It's like saying to my body that I'm not going to be around. So I shifted my thinking. 'Instead, why don't you just pour all your energy into making the time with your kids great, whether it goes on for another thirty years or another seven?' Just be 'that' everyday. Be 'that' loving mother and imprint that in their memories forever and ever, just like the memories I have when I look back to my child-hood and times with my mother as she was a mother to me."

As Karen recovered from her treatment, she grappled with the decision facing most young professional mothers—should she return to work? All of the rationalizations like "I'll be a better mother if I spend some time away from my kids" are more loaded after a cancer diagnosis. When she was first diagnosed, some of her colleagues suggested that she would never come back to work. But this didn't seem right to Karen because she loved her work, worked only half-time, and hadn't found it stressful. She explained the reasoning behind her ultimate decision, "At first I struggled with questions like 'Should I really go back to work?' or 'Shouldn't I just be home with my lap blanket and tell stories to my kids all the time?' And then I realized that if I didn't go back to work, it would be like telling every cell in my body, every part of me, that I only have a few years, and I should just be with the kids. That's not positive at all.

"I only work half-time, so I'm home a lot with them. It's not that I'm a workaholic and they never see me, because I would definitely change if that were the case. So, it's trying to find that balance between living in the moment and planning for the future. I love my job, I'm good at my job, and I get a lot of satisfaction from my job. So it makes sense to me to work.

"I make most of my decisions based on the assumption that I'm going to live. I have found that, in truth, the decisions don't change that much whether I'm going to be around for three years or thirty years. There's a guiding set of values that is the same regardless. That understanding may be one of the blessings of the cancer diagnosis. It helps me to sort out all these decisions."

Even though Karen is able to live her life fully and focus her loving attention on her children, somehow the strategy of focusing on the positive and denying the worries isn't fully working for her. Karen acknowledges that, for some people, living in a form of denial can work well, but she knows she can't do this all the time. She refers to the thought of "dying and leaving my children motherless" as the monster in her subconscious closet.

"There's not a day that goes by that dying doesn't cross my mind—in fact it never really leaves my mind. Even if I try to push it out with a thought blocking technique—such as saying 'Stop that!' every time it might come across my mind—it doesn't work. The thought is still there, somewhere, hidden, and it starts to get a lot of power. Every headache plunges me into fear and despair for three days until it goes away or every ache and pain or every image of a couple growing old with their grandchildren plunges me into negativity. When you're trying not to think about something, you give it more power than it may actually have."

Karen recalled speaking to her minister about her fear of leaving her kids motherless. "At one point he asked, 'What is it about your past experience that tells you that this would be such a devastating thing for your kids?' I was kind of shocked and I could have slapped him. I thought, 'What do you mean? Isn't it obvious? They're losing their mother. Of course it would be devastating. There's no getting around it. There's no 'up' side to it. There's no 'Oh, it might make them closer as siblings.' You just have to acknowledge that it would suck.

"But his question prompted me to explore the possibility that they might still live very fulfilling, very joyful, very rewarding, whole lives— that it wouldn't mean a complete decimation of their world. Yes, if it were to happen, it would be a tragedy and it would be a hardship and it might be the hardest thing that happened in their lives, but they're not going to get through life without hardship.

"For example, it would be the same if you told me my daughter is going to have a stillborn when she's 34 and I might not be there to support her. Am I going to borrow that worry from the future? No, I have to just trust that there would be people there for her like my husband and my sister. I can also trust in their strength.

"I realize that a lot of my feelings about my children losing me as a mother is my own 'trip' of guilt. What if I just died in a car accident quick like that. I would suffer none of this but they would still lose their mother and suffer the same. So I have to realize that some of these emotions are my own baggage."

Karen looks up at the group with resolve. "So when I go into my fear for a while, I'll shine a flashlight at the monster and look at all the nooks and crannies in the closet. And then I'll step back from the monster and think 'Oh, I may not die; and it's not even happening right now; and I might be cured, right?'" A big smile shines through her tears.

By the end of the weekend, having continued to wrestle with the fear of dying young and leaving her kids behind, Karen shared her new perspective with the larger group: "I realize now that it has always been possible for me to die of anything while my children are young and it's always possible for my husband to die too. So, in one sense, nothing magical happened when I discovered I had a serious breast cancer. Nothing momentous changed. I was always a mortal human being who would die at some point.

"The reality now is there is a known threat that may be a little more present and a little more real. It's not a nebulous threat that we can pretend isn't there. So reframing is just realizing that ultimately none of us controls our path in life. There are no guarantees. I could live to 90 and have wasted a decade of my life worrying about what may or may not happen. Or I can live fully and happily to 50 and die of breast cancer. I'd be sad but glad of how I lived the last ten years of my life.

"That's where the choice is; that's where the control is. I don't have control over the ultimate outcome, and I have to accept that. But the most important thing is how I act in this day. I want to be a mother 110 percent every day that I can.

"And that's the gift of getting a cancer diagnosis. It's a slap in the face that says, 'This is your life. It's not a practice run.' From a mothering point of view, I just infuse as much love as I can into every moment because it's in my power to be the best mother I can for today and for tomorrow and for as many tomorrows as I'm given."

CHAPTER 30

Harry and Ann
Living the Tension with Wisdom and Love

Harry is a 64-year-old Saint Nicholas type character with a full beard and a belly laugh to match. He sits beside his wife, Ann, who has been living with an advanced form of a rare cancer called 'carcinoid'.

During the 'Reframing' lecture, Harry reflected on the relationships in his life. His mother died of lung cancer several years ago, at a time when people may not have even mentioned the "C" word. Harry felt badly because he and his mother never really were able to have a frank conversation about how she was feeling. Her only comment to him was that she didn't even want her family to say anything at the memorial service. Harry found the last few weeks with his mother frustrating and unsatisfying. He felt it would have been so much better to have used the time he had to get closer to her.

In contrast, Harry's forty-year marriage with Ann is a full and honest relationship. This is not to say it's always been easy, but Harry shows a remarkable ability to reframe his thinking when times are tough. Harry told his life story as a background to sharing his distressing thoughts in small group discussion.

Harry grew up poor, but considered himself very fortunate. He was a university professor for fifteen years and later directed several charities, retiring five years ago. As a hobby, he now works as a Santa Claus each Christmas, booking gigs and having fun with the kids.

Harry met Ann early in her career as an international development consultant. They traveled widely together, making friends all over the world. They have two grown daughters and are very close as a family.

Ann's lovely character continued to shine even after she developed advanced rheumatoid arthritis, which she's had for thirty years now. Ann discovered there was little support for people affected by arthritis, so she organized the first national conference bringing doctors and patients together. Neither Harry nor Ann thought they would be dealing with another major illness.

Four years ago, cancer came up incidentally at the time of a hysterectomy. Ann's gynecologist noticed a discoloration on Ann's small bowel. An immediate resection of this spot showed that it was a rare tumour called carcinoid that had spread to the abdominal lymph nodes. Fortunately, there was no obvious cancer in other areas of her body and they were told it was a slow growing cancer.

Initially, Ann didn't need any treatment and didn't want to share the diagnosis with her friends. She explained "When you tell people you have cancer, they start treating you differently. They say things like 'Can I get you a chair?' And in the early stages of the disease, that's not appropriate. I'm perfectly capable of getting my own chair."

Harry and Ann decided they could play a role in raising awareness of carcinoid cancer. With her experience as an arthritis advocate, Ann successfully organized a national support group and an annual conference for people with carcinoid tumors. At one point Harry and Ann hosted a regular meeting in their home for eight survivors and their spouses.

Ann wanted to live a normal life, so she continued to work and travel as a consultant for the next three years.

But last year, she developed a growing lump in the skin of her neck. Ann's cancer had recurred in her breast, liver and bone. Ann and Harry began to panic. Compounding the trauma of recurrence was having to deal with the medical system and finding an oncologist with experience with carcinoid cancer.

Initially Ann wasn't covered to see a carcinoid specialist in another province, even though the specialist worked much closer to where they lived. "The medical bureaucracy is quite amazing, so you have to learn, as a patient, what your rights are. For example, we have a complete copy of all of our medical documents, because we keep track of everything that happens. Even with what we have learned, it can be so confusing."

Harry is the information gatherer and chief advocate. He has read a lot about the disease. Ann didn't want to read the articles because she found them depressing. Instead she reads about spiritual concepts and healing journeys, and participates in groups with other women with cancer.

Ann respected her own style of coping. She happily left the medical issues to Harry because she found it too easy to get "sucked into medical solutions or the fears of others." If she was given too much information or was feeling overwhelmed, she would suffer what she calls "sticky brain" which means she would get an idea in her head, and couldn't get rid of it. This made it hard to fall asleep.

Ultimately, Harry and Ann learned that Ann's cancer had mutated into a highly aggressive form and that people with this type of mutation only live an average of six months. On a more positive note, they learned that chemotherapy had an 80 percent chance of shrinking her tumours.

Ann recounts that this was a very trying time in their relationship. "We became very short tempered. We were at each other's throats. The level of stress was extremely high. We were totally focused on cancer. Our daughters were saying, 'Why should we come over and see you when you're so cranky?'" Ann lets out a big laugh reflecting back on the tough times. "I guess we were very unpleasant to be with."

The chemotherapy Ann started six months ago was 'terrible.' A three-week cycle would consist of two weeks of vomiting and diarrhea following by a third week of near normalcy. Before Ann started, she had four carcinoid tumors that were visible on her chest and back. Two months later, there were eleven visible tumors. The doctors agreed the chemotherapy was not working but didn't know what to do next and so suggested palliative care.

Ann continued to work with her mind-body connection. She was excited about our weekend retreat and wanted to learn one or two 'non-aggressive' visualizations for dealing with cancer. She explained, "Most approaches are about fighting against the cancer like it's a war—but that's just not my style. Cancer to me is just a part of my body. I'm an inclusive person, and so I welcome whatever."

A week before the weekend retreat, Ann was scheduled to receive radiotherapy for a spot on her hip. Harry had had trouble adjusting to his changing role during this difficult week. Ann's hip pain had become so intense that she couldn't walk and Harry even had to help her to go to the bathroom. He realized if her legs were to remain weak, their life together would be totally turned upside down. She would not be able to drive any more. He began to contemplate what would happen if she couldn't walk or couldn't take care of herself for the rest of her life.

After several days of radiation, and because of pain and diarrhea, Ann became dehydrated. On the eve of the retreat, she had to be admitted to hospital but, after some intravenous fluids, and through sheer force of will, Ann did join us on Friday evening. By Saturday afternoon, she had to return home to rest, though.

In the small group discussion on "Reframing Distressing Thoughts," Harry felt out of place because Ann had gone home and he was the only person in his group who didn't have a cancer diagnosis. He wondered if he should even be participating in the small group.

The group fell silent after several people had spoken. It was Harry's turn. Harry looked at the sheets he completed during the reframing lecture. He had three full pages of distressing thoughts he's had as a family member, but he didn't feel justified in bringing his concerns to the group. He started, "These thoughts seem very petty compared to the rest of yours."

"I'll just read the ones I don't know how to resolve. My first thought is 'Our retirement plans are ruined, because we can't travel anymore.' I guess that brings out sadness because we had been looking forward to doing things together." He looked to the "reframing" column. "Obviously, there's no real response. We have to find other ways to enjoy our retirement that don't involve international travel. It doesn't entirely resolve the problem of not being able to see our relatives, but we are trying to compensate by phoning, you know, that type of thing."

Harry continued "I had a couple of others: 'I hate to do all the work in the family. It's unfair.'" Harry quickly clarifies this for the group. "Of course, it's not 'all' the work, really, because when she's well she does her share." He laughs to himself and goes on, "Our division of labour is that I've been the cook in our family for about twenty years now and she's the bottle washer. And when I cook I usually make quite a mess in the kitchen; now I have to clean up my own trail of dirty dishes.

"It's even hard to be the cook now. With the cancer, she sometimes doesn't like to eat certain things. She says, 'Well, I can't face meat.' So I said, 'I'll start making vegetarian things.' The first thing I made was two lentil loaves. And she said, 'I don't like them.'" Harry laughed again. "So I had to eat them all. That was a little irritating.

"Here's what I think about it. Life is not fair, and housework is never 100 percent fair, even when both parties are well. I guess what's difficult is when you've been doing things the same way for many years and then you have this change. Your partner can't really do what you counted on them doing in the past, and so you feel kind of like, 'Gee, I have to pick up this, and pick up that, and I have to do this, and all these things I didn't have to do before.' Suddenly you become aware of what your partner did."

Harry let out a big laugh, then added, "I had always wondered who did those various things." The group laughed, but they were struck by Harry's underlying love. They appreciated Harry's honesty in sharing the daily irritations of living in a relationship.

Harry reflected more seriously, "It seems like I'm blaming my wife, but I'm not. I feel a little discouraged. I feel a little resentment. But it's not resentment towards her. It's resentment towards the situation."

Harry went on to his next thought. "'If we have grandchildren, my wife won't know them.' So that's a distressing thought, because our daughters don't have children yet." Harry pauses as he tries to reframe this thought. "I don't see any response to that. It's just a sad element, you know."

Harry did not try to buoy himself up with "Maybe there will be a medical breakthrough, or miracles can always happen." There was no underestimation or exaggeration in this sadness. He has come to an acceptance of the situation. He was choosing not to dwell on this difficult thought, not to continue to feed the flames of sadness, because he didn't want to burn away the precious time they have together.

Harry paused and reflected on his journey. "I ask myself, in this period, 'Am I in touch with my emotions? Am I really seeing the most distressful thoughts that I should be seeing or should I not be seeing them? Should I let them lie where they're at and let them come up when they come up?'

"I don't know. I just try to deal with the situation and not to put ourselves in a funk about things, because it doesn't help your situation to get totally down about it."

Harry also shared his philosophy on how he was trying to look after himself on this journey with Ann. "I realized I had to make some adjustments in my life to take into account Ann's changing health situation. I couldn't go on the way I was going. I've dropped some of my activities, like I dropped out of one of my choirs. But I didn't drop them all, because if I directed all my focus towards the disease, that's not good. I need to keep a positive attitude towards life and keep living. And Ann feels that way too. If I just say 'Woe is me' and let myself get dragged down by the condition, then it is not going to help.

"Like the night before last, I was at the hospital all day with Ann, and it was a terrible day for us. But I went to my barber shop quartet group at night to sing—because I needed to have a little bit of joy that day and to take my mind off our problems."

In the weeks leading up to the retreat, Ann was also living as full a life as she could. Instead of pursuing the chemotherapy that wasn't working, she took painting lessons. She participated in a 5-km walk despite her fatigue. She continued taking singing lessons and had been asked to perform a solo in her church on Easter Sunday.

Ann's legs were weak as she stood before the congregation, but her voice was strong as she sang with heart the hymn by Mendelssohn: "O rest in the Lord, wait patiently for Him, and He shall give thee thy heart's desires, and trust in Him." Ann walked off the stage calmly, her spirit lighting the way for others. Sitting in the pews, Harry worried that this could be Ann's last solo, a prophecy of the months to come.

In the weeks after the solo, Harry could see that Ann was weakening physically. It became more difficult for him to share his feelings. He found it so painful to see Ann get weaker. The retreat turned out to be a place where he could give voice to his greatest fears.

Harry sent the following Christmas email as an account of Ann's remarkable journey. "Just after the retreat, Ann began a sharp physical decline. She had no pain except for one week early on. Mainly her muscles began getting weaker and weaker. With our girls, we took a last family weekend trip to a beautiful resort about one hour from our home where we had, at other critical moments of Ann's illness, made weekend trips for closeness and support. Ann had to use a wheelchair and needed to sleep a lot, but she still managed to enjoy the scenery, good food and family closeness. Although we hoped there would be time for more such outings, I think we each knew, deep inside, that this was to be our last."

Harry could see that Ann was going through the final transition—her inner light was shining more and more brightly as her body began to fade. His email continued, "Finally she was bed-ridden and, since she had decided she wanted to die at home, we had a hospital bed brought in so she could look out the window at the flowers and so we could better care for her.

"All through the last year, Ann had a care team from the church come in to help her—all women, all very different people. They were just great. Sitting with her, reading to her, talking to her, and bringing us food. Such loving care. I can never repay that.

"It was tough emotionally to have such a strong woman become so weak. I brought her a drink with a straw and she couldn't even sip. I felt so powerless and I wanted to cry.

"For the last three days, we had the help of a night nurse who specializes in hospice care to guide us and enable us to get some sleep. We spent a lot of time with Ann, played beautiful music, and talked with and to her. It was, in many ways, a beautiful period of our lives although, of course, very sad also. We were grateful that Ann had virtually no pain in the lead up to her death. We were also grateful for her attitude—she was courageous and accepted her impending death.

"On the day Ann died, the nurse woke us at 2:00 AM to say that Ann had lost consciousness and was close to death. We played soft music and sang to her. We held her hand. She died at noon, with our love surrounding her. Sarah, my daughter, gave her a final bath. The girls wanted to keep her at the house for a few hours before starting the funeral home arrangements.

"We would have celebrated our fortieth year of marriage a month later. Ann was a wonderful wife and mother and we all miss her dearly."

Ann always wanted to share her story with others because she wanted to raise awareness of carcinoid tumors.

She was a great teacher. Even in the dying process, she was the light of peace and love. Sadly, Ann didn't live long enough to hear that her daughter Sarah was pregnant. Ann really wanted to be a grandmother.

Ann's deep love, compassion for others, and generosity of spirit connected her to everyone in her life. Ann's inner light will continue to shine on in Harry, her two daughters, her granddaughter, and the many others she touched.

Reclaiming
Our Wholeness

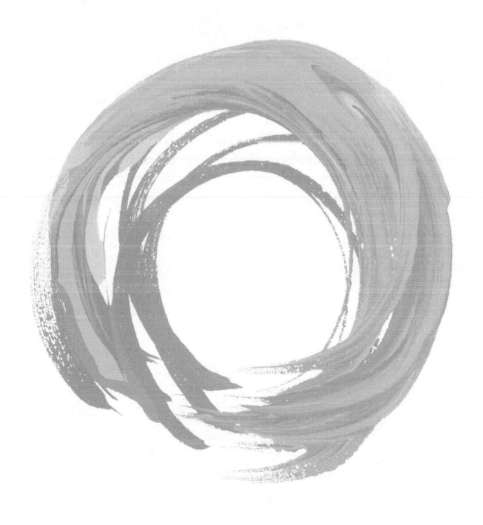

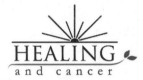
and cancer

Sunday • Reclaiming our Wholeness

In this section of the book, you will listen to the Sunday morning talks and discussions which demonstrate that loss, anxiety, grief, and anger have many lessons to teach us. You will also hear stories about people who were able to honour their difficult emotions, and transform their fear of dying into their joy of living.

As you shine light into the dark spaces of your psyche you will find that all experiences are workable and no aspect of your being ever needs to be rejected. Looking at your fears directly and embracing all of your emotions, you can free your life energy to flow through you and heal your life at a deeper level.

The journey of reclaiming your already existing wholeness is a journey of bringing together body, emotions, mind and spirit to help you to see yourself from the vast perspective of the inner and outer circles of life.

To view the touching short documentary about Julie and Randy (the subject of chapter 40) visit the 'video' link at www.HealingandCancer.org

CHAPTER 31

The Bowl of Loving Kindness Meditation

Love and compassion, the open path, is associated with "what is." In order to develop love - universal love, cosmic love, whatever you would like to call it - one must accept the whole situation of life as it is, both the light and the dark, the good and the bad. One must open oneself to life, and communicate with it.

Chogyam Trungpa

Sunday morning. *The people at the retreat, most of whom had never met each other two days before, are now warmly chatting and sipping their tea or coffee. Peals of laughter spill from the hallway while some couples sit close beside each other holding hands, talking or smiling in silence.*

Everyone, to their own degree of comfort, has gradually opened up to others, to themselves, and to the larger group as a whole. Like removing their winter coats, scarves, and hats, each person, in their own way, has exposed the tender sweetness of who they are, and revealed their tremendous courage, and shared their inner struggles. Through their openness, the healing circle is becoming a living, breathing reality.

Tim leads the group in the opening meditation of the day which foreshadows the profound work of transforming the darkest and most difficult emotions. People in the circle drop into silence, taking the posture for meditation, and listen to and follow these instructions.

The Bowl of Loving Kindness Meditation

Hands resting gently on your knees or thighs
Lift your heart just a little bit towards the sky
Tuck your chin a little bit
Open the crown of your head up to the sky above
Make contact with the earth below
At the same time begin to open up the upper body
To make a connection with the sky,
Connecting to the vastness of the universe

In our bodies we join those energies of the heaven above
With the solid grounded energy of earth below
Let your body become a conduit or conductor
Being mindful of each breath
Bringing yourself into total presence
Be fully in the here and now

Honour and feel that life force that pulses in the body
Really feel that inner field of energy

From this place of openness and presence
We will begin a guided visualization........

Slowly and mindfully turn your hands upward on your lap
Now, imagine that you're holding a bowl in your lap
A beautiful large bowl resting in your hands
You can design this bowl however you like
It can be organic or magical, made of wood or stone
Or beautiful luminous glass, or made of pure energy
And beautiful coloured light
Admire its beauty
Then once again tuning into your heart
The energetic heart center in the middle of your chest
Find that place that naturally glows with the light of loving kindness
This heart center is like a receiver and transmitter of the universal energy of love,
healing and creative transformation
Allow your heart to warm up and begin to glow

Like the light of the sun rising in the morning
As that light radiates, sending healing light to every cell of your body
It also spills its healing energy out of your heart and into the bowl in your lap
Gradually the bowl fills up and becomes radiant with the light of loving kindness

Gently raise the corners of the mouth ever so slightly
Into a gentle little smile of peace and simple joy
Notice how that affects the feeling in your body
Something begins to shift in your inner being
Bringing a little smile into your energy body
Now bring that smile into your heart
As if you could smile from your heart
Then allow that smile to radiate from your heart into the bowl
Filling the bowl with the light of loving kindness
Watch as the pure light swirls and sparkles in the bowl

Now search deep within to find all of those difficult emotions
Fear, anger, impatience, frustration, any sense of hopelessness or despair,
You begin to pour these one by one or place them into the bowl
Pull all the so-called negative emotions out of your system wherever they reside
Searching into any of the dark, hidden corners of your being
Anger, fear, self-pity, guilt, self-hatred and judgments of all kinds
Feeling inadequate or insecure, feeling unworthy, or not being good enough
A sense of not belonging, feeling unlovable,
Confusion and despair, all the many difficult and painful emotions
Whatever you have the hardest time with, put it into the bowl
And then again radiate the light of loving kindness from your heart
The unconditional, universal power of love that naturally radiates
And again, fill the bowl with loving kindness

As you do, watch those energies mix
Watch how the energy of loving kindness flows
And mixes with the energy of your difficult emotions
The energy of feeling unworthy
The impatience and fear
Allow those energies to mix with the light of loving kindness
The light of loving kindness penetrates into the hardness of these emotions
Breaking them up and dissolving them back into pure energy

Watch as the lights begin to swirl and mix together
Into a beautiful swirling mix of colors
All of those difficult feelings can be transformed
Back into the pure energy of life itself
Don't leave any behind in your system
Pour them all in to be transformed and mixed with loving kindness
All of your own unique difficulties
Recognize them, call them out, and put them out in front of you
Mixing them with light of loving kindness
Radiate that light from your heart
Saying 'I love and accept myself exactly as I am
All of my feelings, all of my energy'
Mix those feelings with love, acceptance and peace
Now look into that bowl and see the swirling beauty of lights
Transformation and acceptance

Then, when you're ready
Bring that bowl slowly up and into your heart
Gently lift that bowl raising your hands up
And place your hands on your chest gently over your heart
Dissolving the bowl and all that good energy back inside yourself
Feel that richness and fullness of it all
Universal purity
Life-giving healing energy flows into your body, into your being, into your psyche

Then, when you're ready, dissolve the visualization
And put your hands back gently on your knees or thighs
Allow your mind to dissolve into a clear blue sky
Opening your mind, expanding into the vastness of space
Feeling grounded on the earth
Connecting with your breath
And feeling that sense of life
Awake and alert and energized
Feel your feet on the floor
Sitting bones on the seat
Head and shoulders reaching to the sky
Smile and enjoy this moment
When you are ready bring your attention back
And be here now

This guided meditation is like the alchemical work of old, where contemplative masters worked to transform the "lead" of their conflicting emotions and distorted thoughts into the "gold" of wisdom, compassion, and healing. The alchemists had a container into which they put the base substances to be transformed. The container gave them a little bit of distance and detachment from their normal experience of holding emotions. Then with a secret and magical process that involved heat and light, they would transform or *transmute* these base substances into pure gold.

We, too, can engage in this process and follow the path of transforming emotions. We can think of this magical process as our meditative concentration and the heat and light as our ability to tap into the power of loving kindness which is always available to us. The container in this visualization is the bowl, but ultimately it is also our full and open heart and the openness of our physical body to accommodate and enjoy the power of our emotional energy and spirit.

There is an important wisdom teaching embedded in this visualization. It is connected with acknowledging and learning to access our inherent wholeness and goodness. The wisdom is to simply know and to experience that the energy of our difficult and painful emotions is actually *good* energy, and that given the right approach and the right conditions, this energy can be redirected into healing and into compassion toward ourselves and others.

CHAPTER 32

Peter
Letting Anger Come

"It wasn't until Friday night that I realized how angry I was."

Peter is the first person to take the microphone during the Sunday morning check-in. He is a strapping, handsome 37-year old man, with dark brown eyes and black hair, and his voice has a lovely pitch, lilting with what sounds like an Irish accent. His face is serious as he looks to the group, turning occasionally, as if for reassurance, to his wife sitting beside him. Janet, a beautiful young woman in the midst of chemotherapy, smiles at him, her eyes crinkling at the edges from under a bright polka-dot hat.

"On Friday night, Janet and I fought all the way home in the car. And it's a forty minute drive."

Janet had convinced Peter to come to the retreat with her, hoping they would both learn some skills to help cope with their difficult situation. Knowing his wife typically knew what was best, Peter agreed, but found himself increasingly irritated during the evening as he listened to many stories of people who weren't as sick as Janet.

"That was a total waste of time," he told Janet in the car. "What's the point of going to a retreat?" Long silences were interspersed with spats about little things. When they got home, Janet kissed their boys, aged 7 and 10, and put them to bed. She then asked Peter to come to bed with her as she was tired from the long day. Peter snapped, "It's too early to go to bed. I'm going to watch television!"

Peter didn't make it to the TV. Instead he sat alone in the darkness of his den, gritting his teeth, stewing over the evening. In the silence, he heard a kinder voice gently whisper, "Why am I like this? Why am I being rude to Janet, a woman I deeply love and respect and who has been joined to me for over half of my life?" He knew he wasn't mad at Janet…it was something else, something percolating deep within. As he pondered, images of their life together began to flow across his mind.

They had met when they were both 19, and began to live together when Janet went to college and Peter worked as a lumberjack, cutting down trees and chain sawing them into 8-foot lengths. By the time they married at age 24, Janet worked as a teller in the bank and Peter was start-ing to question whether he wanted to work in the woods for the rest of his life.

Two years later their first son was born, and family and church became the focus of their lives. Seeing that Peter wasn't happy, Janet kept encour-aging him to do something else. She believed in him, knowing his natural intelligence and kind way with people would make him a success no matter where he went. But even after their second boy was born, Peter still persisted in doing heavy labour in the woods until a tree fell on him and crushed his ribs. Alone in the woods, in severe pain, he crawled on his hands and knees for two miles to the closest truck. When he finally got home, Janet took one look at him and exclaimed "Enough! You're going back to school."

At age 30, setting aside their concerns about finances, Peter enrolled in a degree program in nursing. He was a natural, with a quick-wit and good natured disposition. The regional hospital quickly snapped him up when he finished his studies.

Life was great. The boys were happy, active in baseball and hockey, thriving in school, and fed with the loving attention of their mother. Even when Janet had to have a small portion of her bowel removed for a benign tumour, they were grateful for everything they had. Peter grinned thinking how he joked with Janet when her surgery date landed on their 10th' wedding anniversary, "Going to the hospital was probably just how she felt on the day she married me. A little bit sick!"

Upon graduating, Peter chose to work in palliative care. Meanwhile, in spite of her previous bowel surgery, Janet was troubled by worsening cramps in her pelvis which her doctors couldn't explain. One afternoon, Janet lay grimacing, curled up in bed, but insisted that Peter go in to work as Peter's mother would be taking care of the kids.

The next morning, Peter returned home from his night shift to a shocking sight. Janet's abdomen had ballooned and she was as white as a ghost. As Peter rushed downstairs to call an ambulance, Janet weakly called out "Don't call them. I need to get dressed." Peter shouted back, "Are you crazy? You could die any minute and you want to look good?"

But Janet, a strong woman even when ill, persuaded Peter to drive her to the hospital. A CAT scan showed a mass in her ovary and blood in her abdomen. Emergency surgery ensued, followed by a horrible wait for the results: Janet had a very slow-growing type of tumour called carcinoid that had spread from the small bowel to the ovary. Even though all the visible cancer had been resected, her doctors recommended that Janet start on chemotherapy.

Peter remembers that the specialists tried to encourage them saying Janet's cancer was slow-growing, non-aggressive, and easily treated. They told Peter and Janet that most people with carcinoid live for more than 10-15 years, adding "If you're going to have cancer, this is the one to have."

To Peter, the news and their words weren't reassuring. And sadly, the doctors were wrong in their predictions. It seemed that every medical appointment was met with more bad news. Six months after Janet's first chemotherapy, a scan showed the cancer had spread to a spot in her liver. After a resection of this tumor, a spot showed up in her stomach wall. Most recently, the tumour was back again in multiple spots in the liver, growing faster than ever expected.

Worse still, the chemotherapy pills caused Janet to be nauseated, forcing her on some days to choose between staying on a regimen that might extend her life, or skipping the pills so she could enjoy the time with her young boys. Janet's strong faith in God helped make this whole ordeal easier for everyone. She would say "I try to give it to God. Because it's out of my control, there's nothing I can do about it. And that gives me comfort." She prayed to find the strength to make their family life as normal as possible, because she didn't want her kids to miss out on a happy childhood.

Peter sat in his den thinking about how unfair this all was. This beautiful woman had done nothing to deserve such a bad fate. As waves of anger washed over him, he did nothing to stop the feelings that were bubbling up.

Peter thought about all the people who helped them through this awful situation. At first, the outpourings of generosity were overwhelming and almost made him feel helpless, which was hard for him to accept as a man. Casseroles and unsigned gift cards would show up on the front porch. The driveway would be ploughed without explanation. The phone just never stopped ringing. The kids would be whisked away to hockey practice as if by magic. People he knew by face only would tap him on the shoulder at the end of Mass and tell him that they would pop by later that day with a 'little something.' Peter smiled to himself, "They say you can't see angels – but we see them every day, coming to our door with something...they are definitely angels, sent by God."

Peter was frustrated at times, thinking he should be able to handle their family problems by himself. But with a large student loan, Janet off work, and Peter home taking care of her, he needed to refinance their mortgage to deal with growing debts. One afternoon, on a cold winter's day, when they were flat broke and the mortgage payment was overdue, there was a knock at the door. There stood Roberta, a nurse from Peter's work. Handing over an envelope with $1200 collected from the hospital staff, this small woman gave Peter a hug, and turned and walked away.

They continued to manage somehow, making ends meet, keeping the boys active. Peter and Janet enjoyed their walks along the lake whenever they could and would talk about everything, including writing a will for Janet. They were honest with each other and their emotions. Their mottos were to 'Cry today, and fight the cancer tomorrow.' and 'Live with it, but don't dwell on it.'

But they also had their disagreements and difficult times. For example, as it became more obvious that Janet was going to die of her cancer, both he and Janet had stopped talking about their greatest fears and the grief that was smouldering inside. During their 'big silence', Peter could feel mounting irritation with the world, and began to admit to himself how much stress he was feeling.

Being a palliative care nurse made being his role as husband more complicated. In Peter's work world, he was expected to be positive, despite the extreme difficulties his patients were going through. He also expected to be in control at work and to know what to do in almost every situation. At home, he tried to stay positive all the time, but that meant he was hiding his true feelings. Also he had to admit he couldn't control everything.

Peter remembered one evening when Janet's nausea had peaked and her gut was aching. Frustrated at seeing her suffering, Peter insisted that Janet try an IV medication, and he would start one for her. But Janet shook her head "I don't want you to be my nurse, I want you to be my husband!"

Other images from working on the palliative care ward came to Peter's mind. A young woman, surrounded by her family died without pain, and in some way seemed to shine with her final breaths. Sitting in the darkness, Peter thought "I hope Janet can have a peaceful death." He stopped himself in mid-breath. A surge of guilt rushed in as a second inner voice asked "How can you even think like that? Do you want to rush her death thinking about the future?"

The thoughts, feelings and fears that had plagued him for months kept popping to mind, one after the other. "What should we be telling the kids right now?...Should they go visit her in the hospital when she's about to die?...How am I ever going to tell them when she dies?... How do I tell my mother?... How do I tell everyone else?"

Peter, already choked up, then heard his greatest fears come to mind: "How could I ever fill that void? How can I even raise our kids - I can't even dress them right!" He remembers Janet's reaction one night, from her hospital bed, on hearing that Peter had put one of the boys in an old pair of jeans and bright green shirt "You didn't send him to school like that, did you?" He shakes his head in the darkness "She'll always thinking about what's best for them."

By now, Peter's tears had begun to flow freely as he sat in his den, in the dark.

His many feelings, of helplessness, of fear of the unknown, and of anger, could no longer be suppressed.

He resolved to be more honest with himself and with Janet and to seek professional help to work through the grief he was suffering.

By Sunday morning he was ready to share his insights with the group during the check-in. "Like I said, it wasn't until Friday night that I realized how angry I was. When we left here, I'm telling you, we fought all the way home. I complained about everything. But I didn't really understand what was going on inside me and it wasn't until later that night, after Janet had gone to bed, that it finally hit me. I'm so mad because this isn't fair for her, it's not fair for our children. It's not fair for any of us. We had plans and dreams and cancer changed everything. But I can't believe that it wasn't until Friday night that I realized how mad I was about the whole thing.

"I think I've told myself all along, 'Well, you shouldn't be angry, that's not a good emotion, right? You shouldn't be angry, that won't help anyone.' But I was angry, and I am angry. And hiding it inside doesn't work either. I think that's a big thing that's come up for me this weekend, that it's okay to be angry, it's okay to be down, it's okay to feel whatever you feel. I think trying to pretend it's not there has caused a lot of tension between us.

"I didn't even want to come here this weekend but I guess Janet knew what was best for me. The whole retreat has been an environment where I can express myself freely. I've felt that I'm with others who could understand."

Janet nods emphatically in agreement. Peter goes on. "I had this anger and I've been short and frustrated, because I don't think I ever really dealt with it. I'm supposed to be the nurse, right? I'm supposed to help people and I thought to do that I had to just stuff my anger inside. Now I know I have to learn to be with it. Now, it makes so much sense, because when you suppress it…"

Janet jumps in here, completing her husband's sentence: "…it's not really gone; it just keeps coming back."

Peter looks at Janet with a twinkle in his eyes. "Yeah, and it comes out in weird ways with you and the kids. But when I really accept the anger, like on Friday night, I can work through it and see that it is not so bad. I can handle it, without blowing up, right?"

Janet nods and smiles.

CHAPTER 33

Embracing Emotions
with Kindness and Awareness

The spiritual journey involves going beyond hope and
fear, stepping into unknown territory, and continually
moving forward. The most important aspect of being
on the spiritual path may be to just keep moving.
Usually, when we reach our limit, we freeze in terror.
Ourbodies freeze and so do our minds. Rather than
indulge or reject our experience, we can somehow let
the energy of the emotion, the quality of what we're
feeling pierce us to the heart. This is a noble way to live.
It's the path of compassion – the path of cultivating
human bravery and kind-heartedness.
Pema Chrödrön

Sunday morning. *After opening meditation and Peter's story, Tim draws on
his experience as a psychotherapist and spiritual teacher, to encourages people to
embrace all their emotions.*

The mindful and open-hearted approach of the weekend retreat is not
about making all of life's difficulties go away. Reframing distressing
thoughts can help put life in perspective and will definitely lessen emotional turmoil but we are still bound to feel angry, scared, depressed and
just plain awful at times. Emotions have a raw and energetic quality, and
can be embraced. We can honour this energy as part of the natural human
experience. Learning how to work directly with the energy of emotions
is helpful in reclaiming our wholeness.

The word emotion comes from the Latin root-word *emovare* which means 'to move out' and is also the root word of 'motivate' and 'motivation'. Movement is the essential nature of emotions as we can let them move through our bodies in a healthy way and out into the world through our words and actions. In this sense, we can think of emotions as energy in motion.

Think back to a hot and muggy summer day. The atmosphere is thick with moisture pressing on your body and it's like breathing in hot soup. Suddenly in the late afternoon, lightning flashes, illuminating everything in brilliant contrasts; thunder rolls, reverberating in your body; and a fresh rain pours down from high above. The humidity and the temperature drop all at once. After a while, just as quickly as it came, the storm breaks up, clouds part and the sun shines again.

Emotions flow and change like the weather. Emotional storms can happen in the atmosphere of our relationships with family members and friends and in our relationship with ourselves. The emotional atmosphere can become hot and muggy as tensions build and are not addressed. Suddenly something will trigger a dramatic deluge and release built up pressure. After the storm there can be a clearing and a freshness. We are now in a different place and can acknowledge, with hindsight, that there was a storm brewing all along.

Elizabeth Kubler-Ross described the stages of grief in dealing with loss in her classic book *On Death and Dying*. She explained that facing loss and drastic changes in our lives will naturally bring up strong and painful emotions, and that most people go through the emotional stages of denial, anger, bargaining or magical thinking, depression and acceptance.

These stages of grief are just a guideline though, as some people go through the stages in a different order, or they may skip a stage, or blend two stages together or repeat others. Nonetheless, these stages are a helpful guidepost as we observe ourselves and understand it is normal to have these strong and shifting feelings.

Just as the sun warms the earth, creating global weather patterns and distinct climates, so life energy flows in our environment, in our relationships, around us, and into our bodies. This life energy, shaped by the complex patterns in our thoughts, our intentions and our relationships, becomes emotions and this energy can sometimes become blocked.

From the perspective of viewing emotions as the flowing energy of our life we can think of Kubler-Ross' progression of stages as a way learning to flow with reality rather than obstructing the truth of life's dramatic changes. As long as we do not deny the flow of our emotional energy, our inner and outer barometric pressure can be synchronized so that big walls of pressure do not build up.

Denial takes on many forms from the initial shock and not truly believing the cancer diagnosis to longstanding problems of denying one's anger or other authentic feelings. In all situations of denial, we have unconsciously or consciously decided we are not going to fully believe what is happening. We are deliberately blocking the truth of the situation because it is just too painful. This is a very natural reaction in the case of a cancer diagnosis.

However, while in denial, emotions can become frozen or continue to surface unpredictably. On the outside we may be putting on a good show for our loved ones or even for ourselves, but the underlying emotions can become stuck some place inside of us. When that raw life force energy becomes dammed up, our true emotions stop flowing.

Unblocking Emotions

So if emotions are energy in motion, then how do they get stuck and how do we encourage them to flow in a healthy way? We have already learned how distressing and irrational thoughts can create painful emotions and depressed states. When our thoughts are inaccurate and out of touch with reality, we can find ourselves spinning our wheels, recycling the same emotional reactions over and over.

When we get stuck in a certain way of repetitive thinking, our emotions also get entangled in that thought structure. In other words, our emotions follow the pathways created by our thoughts. If our thoughts are stuck, they can block our emotional energy.

Many of us have been systematically trained not to feel what we are in fact feeling. Due to social, cultural, and family pressures, we often think "I shouldn't be feeling this way" and we then try to shut the feeling down. Children hear "Don't feel bad; don't be angry; don't be sad; don't cry; don't get so excited; don't upset your mother; don't speak to your father that way…" and countless other emotional suppressants, thousands of times over the years of growing up. As a result, most of us have developed some form of coping mechanism that involves suppressing what we are truly feeling or we pretend to feel one way when, in truth, we are feeling another. The opposite of suppressing emotions is acting out emotions when we simply explode outward with their life force energy, often in very childish ways that wreak havoc in our relationships.

The good news is that there is another way. There is a *middle* way of working with our emotions, a mature and intelligent way, between acting them out and suppressing them. The 'middle way' option, to avoid falling into either of these two extremes, is to be mindfully present to our feelings as they arise, to simply feel them, and then eventually to transform the energy and put it to good use.

For instance, one person, in her small group, described having an awful time getting through chemotherapy because of all the side effects she was suffering. It was normal for her to feel angry and frustrated with all this. However, suppressing her frustration because she thought she shouldn't feel angry just caused more stress. Alternatively, acting out her anger by yelling at her doctors or her husband wasn't helping anyone.

A healthy, middle way is for her to feel her anger and to express it honestly with someone who can hear her, or to focus that energy into an exercise program, or to breathe through her anger and discover the intelligence in it. This practice of holding or experiencing emotions in our bodies, with mindfulness and awareness, can bring about a natural healing process, but is often very difficult to do.

Why We Have Difficulty Experiencing Our Emotions

People often find experiencing their emotions difficult for several reasons. One reason is that it goes against the way they have been taught and how they have managed their feelings since they were children. In other words, it goes counter to the "emotional software" that they have become habituated to in their life.

If we are to change these old patterns, we need first to recognize them. By practicing mindfulness, we can be fully present to these patterns, without bias or judgement. Through awareness, we can begin to see and feel that these old patterns (like suppression or acting out) cause us excess grief. This awareness leads to a greater wisdom that can gradually transform our way of being with our emotions.

A second reason that we find it sometimes difficult to simply be with our feelings is that we literally have a hard time holding the energy in our body. Think for a moment about what it is like when you are very angry and you are doing your very best not to blow up or act out your anger. You may have felt your body heating up, getting 'hot under the collar'. As you hold back from shouting or lashing out, your body might even shake with the power of all that emotional energy held in so tightly. As one woman explained, "It is like my whole body is electrified or something. All of a sudden I feel like every nerve in my body has just been lit up like a Christmas tree. It is electrifying. I can feel it right down into my hair follicles."

When feelings are very strong or unfamiliar to us, we literally don't have the channels and pathways or the capacity to hold that energy in our body. As my healing teacher, Jason Shulman, likes to say, "We need to learn to grow our container." It is possible to learn on a very physical and visceral level to expand our ability to contain and channel these powerful emotional energies. Mindfulness-based stress reduction, belly breathing and the body scan, with practice, can transform your body so the energy flows in a more free and healthy way. Meditation, yoga, martial arts, Qi Gong, and Tai Chi can also be extremely helpful in slowly transforming your physical body into a larger, more open container for the powerful flowing energy of your emotions.

Distorted Thinking about Emotions

We also tend to carry some pretty funny belief patterns, unquestioned, under the surface of our thoughts, about *how* to work with our emotions. One such belief goes something like this: "Someday I am going to work it all out, then I won't be going through these emotional ups and downs, then everything will be just fine." We think we are going to miraculously find some steady state where we won't have to experience the 'negative emotions.' Though this is a very common way of thinking, it is actually an irrational and distorted thought, similar to the magical thinking of childhood. Life will have its ups and downs and feelings will also naturally come and go.

By practicing mindfulness meditation we begin to notice all of these magical ways of thinking, and then let them go and come back to reality. With practice we learn to embrace the peaks and valleys of our emotional life with gentleness and a sense of humour. We learn through observation of emotions that every arrival is the beginning of a new departure. We learn to be comfortable that there is no steady state in life. We grow wise.

Another notion that many people hold is "There is a right way to navigate the emotional journey and there is a wrong way, and I am going to do it right." This way of thinking causes one to judge oneself and try to control and shape what is a flowing process. There is no 'right way' and the key is to let our emotional energy flow and unfold in its own unique way, based on who we are, where we have come from, the life we have lived, and what we have learned so far. There is no point in *judging* our approach as right or wrong. When we judge or try to fit ourselves into a frozen model, we tend to stay stuck. With mindful observation we will learn, grow and heal.

Healing through Emotions

Learning to work with and transform the energy of emotions is an essential step on the healing journey. The energy of thoughts and emotions, our psychological realm of experience, is the life-force energy that links our physical body to the realm we might refer to as spiritual, a realm beyond thoughts and concepts. The energy of emotions can be like the lightning bolts that join together heaven and earth in a thunder storm.

There is wisdom in the energy of your emotions that is simple and direct. Emotions are a human way of experiencing the life force energy, your very life and vitality. This elemental wisdom joins body mind and spirit together into a unified whole and connects you in a direct way to your environment.

We tend to think of our bodies as solid matter bound in space and ending at the place where skin meets the air. On the energetic level, however, the concepts of inside and outside do not apply in the same way. Think about how the words you speak when you are angry can go straight into the emotional brain of your partner, igniting an intense reaction. Emotional energy definitely flows between people. This means that loving kindness and compassion can also flow and circulate in a circle of healing.

In the example of working with the flow of anger above, each person can learn to take full responsibility for how they shape and work with this energy. When we are mindful of the words we use to express our anger as well as mindful of our reactions to another's anger, then the anger itself can become a powerful force for change in the relationship. When both people learn to listen to one another, to respect one another, and communicate in a way that allows both people to get their needs met. The relationship can function more openly and honestly.

The free flow of life energy in our system is what we experience as being alive. Think back for a moment to a time when you felt very alive. Chances are, you felt very connected to the people and natural environment around you. Now think of a time when you felt unwell, depressed or somehow stuck. Chances are you felt separated from your environment and the people in your life.

Good health is actually very dependent upon the free flow of life energy. In Traditional Chinese Medicine and Qi Gong, the free movement of energy in and around the body is seen as a significant variable underlying health and happiness.

When you hold yourself with loving kindness, you make some mental and emotional breathing space for yourself, and there is room for your emotions to flow. Then it is possible to learn from your experience and to change, grow and transform. When you don't "try too hard" to get it right, when you allow for mistakes and use each mistake as a stepping stone, then learning unfolds naturally and progress towards embracing wholeness is inevitable.

When you can relax your body with belly breathing and simply observe the sensations of your emotions without getting caught up in thoughts about the emotions, then the energy in the emotions naturally resolves itself. That energy becomes available to use in your life to enhance your sense of well-being, your vitality, and confidence. With consistent awareness emotional energy can be transformed into compassion, love and gratitude and then channelled into healing and joyful living.

To begin to heal, simply listen to your feelings and honour them just as they are. Using mindfulness meditation, allow yourself to be still and quiet, to follow the breath, and train yourself not to get lost in the tangle of your thoughts. Over time, you will learn to observe the inner weather of your emotions, without judging, without suppressing, and without acting out. As you liberate bound up energy, you will facilitate your own healing in the circles of energy that flow between body, mind and spirit.

CHAPTER 34

Jackie
From a Closed Hand to an Open Hand

"Four years ago, I found this lump in my breast and it was cancer. My first thought was, 'I'm going to die.' And my second thought was, 'The world is going to fall apart because I'm not going to be there to run it.'" Jackie laughs warmly at herself, her hazel eyes sparkling as she speaks. A bubbly woman in her early forties, she is the 'supermom' of a family of five children and worked as a psychology assistant before her diagnosis.

Jackie's wise and vulnerable nature made her a magnet to many at work and in her church community, as she did her best to "take care of everyone and everything." When she got sick, though, she had to walk away from her contract work which, in turn, caused financial stresses for Jackie and her husband. Jackie's extended family was happy to send them money every month. Her friends from church organized shopping and food, delivering a neatly-wrapped dinner every night during chemotherapy. Jackie felt surrounded by love and willingly handed over the tight control she had on her life. Her trust in her friends and her oncologist was complete.

After almost a year of surgery, chemotherapy and radiation, the monthly financial contributions stopped and the care packages soon disappeared. Life was 'back to normal' but Jackie somehow felt that even though her physical treatments were over, she was just at the beginning of her recovery. Still exhausted from chemotherapy, and trying to run her family again, she would wake up in the middle of night, heart pounding, with the fear of dying gnawing at her.

Anxiety had plagued Jackie since childhood. As a young mother her greatest fear was that one of her kids would die or that she'd die and leave them motherless. In her mind she was now living in this nightmare.

Two years after the original diagnosis, Jackie's cancer recurred in her bones. She told each of her kids in turn that she would restart chemotherapy and she was not expecting to be cured. Hearing this news, her daughter, Sophie, began to sob and sob. Jackie held Sophie in her arms, allowing her child to express the depths of her pain. Jackie reflected later,

"It was really healthy for Sophie to bawl her eyes out. When I'm able to simply be present, I feel like I'm helping my children grieve my death while I'm still alive. That's being the best mom I can be. As awful as that was, I learned I could do it."

Jackie was drawn back into the medical system, looking for answers that weren't there. Well-intentioned friends would share articles and websites of the latest treatments and alternative medicines. One friend even asked Jackie if she'd like to meet a woman with incurable cancer who was flying to Cuba every three months for scorpion venom injections.

Jackie declined but still stewed over whether she was doing everything possible to help herself. Eventually she learned to let go of these worries by praying: "God, I just can't figure out what I should do. If I need to look into scorpion venom, you're going to have to send me a sign." And then she simply would let it go.

Instead of worrying, Jackie launched herself on her own healing journey, exploring all types of complementary medicine and healing techniques, willing to do the hard work of spiritual growth. On Mondays, she'd go to Yoga and pottery. On Tuesday mornings, she attended the local cancer support centre's meditation class. Tuesday afternoon, a friend gave her an individualized Pilate's lesson in her home. Tuesday night was choir, and on Wednesday, she'd collapse for a day. Thursday morning started with Tai Chi and in the afternoon Jackie attended a support group and would see her spiritual advisor. She did yoga and meditation every morning, was on a reducing diet, swam and walked her dog.

Between all of this and taking care of her kids, she also set aside quiet time every day. "From noon till three, I tell people not to phone me. That's my time. I have a self hypnosis tape that my naturopath gave me or sometimes I have a nap if I'm tired. I also try to write in my journal and I pray every day." Jackie stops to reflect on everything she was doing and bursts into laughter. "You know what I am?" She pauses with a chuckle. "I'm an over-achiever!"

At the core of her healing journey is a deep-rooted faith in God. Every Sunday morning Jackie sits in the pews and opens her heart to her Heavenly Father. In the first years after the cancer diagnosis, she'd ask God why she got cancer, feeling sorry for herself, crushed by the sense of loss and unfairness.

Jackie began to seek guidance from Sister Martha, one of the spiritual directors at her church, to deal with her emotional torment. One day,

Sister Martha suggested that Jackie allow herself to experience these difficult feelings fully.

The following Sunday, at the start of Lent, Jackie got the strong sense that God wanted her to follow through on Sister Martha's suggestion. Jackie's first thought was "God, are you nuts? This is going to be messy." Upon reflection, Jackie decided to take God up on the invite and to experience her feelings fully rather than ignoring or avoiding them.

The next three days were intense as she let herself cry at will. Everything went wrong. The drywaller didn't show up during a critical part of renovations; the kids were going rangy, stuck inside during April showers. Jackie would go up to her room and cry for an hour. After her strongest emotions passed she would practice a breathing exercise, write in her journal, or pray. Then she would return to the chaos of family life.

Jackie continued to struggle with her faith and wanted proof that God loved and supported her. While Sister Martha listened intently to her concerns, it often felt to her that God would come into the room, as if a third person was present. Jackie then understood it was her choice to open to Divine Presence, or not, in any situation.

During weekly meetings with Sister Martha, Jackie continued to express her worries about death or whether God really loved her – struggling with these same issues again and again. Seeing that Jackie was judging herself for not making progress on her spiritual path, Sister Martha suggested that her journey is like a spiral. Although Jackie kept coming back to the same issues, she would be on a different level each time. With each pass she could more closely approach the core of her fears. Jackie likens this process to 'growing down'. She explains "I just love babies. They are such perfect little people. As babies grow up though, life just puts on more and more layers of armour on them. And I'm getting to a part in my life where I'm starting to grow down - taking off the layers and approaching the center of the spiral."

Sister Martha's and Jackie's conversations were not restricted to profound spiritual questions. At one point Jackie had gained ten pounds due to a side effect of chemotherapy and her inability to exercise. She knew it was ridiculous to worry about her appearance in the midst of a life-threatening illness. With further reflection she realized her judgment stemmed from her fear of being accepted and the belief that life would be 'crappy' unless she actively worked to make it good.

Through this struggle Jackie felt God was teaching her to accept herself and that life is good even in the midst of difficulties. She was being asked to let go of her fears about her weight. "I just learned to trust that it will all be okay and I'm not going to turn into a 300 pound person. I just had to let it go."

The issue of letting go of judgments from others peaked when Jackie found herself restricted to a wheelchair for a period of a few months. Her oncologist found a chemotherapy that kept her liver spots in check but unfortunately the drug caused a blistering rash on her hands and feet. Jackie was forced to stay off her feet to prevent the breakdown of her skin but the wheelchair presented a problem for walking her Newfoundland dog, Daphne.

Jackie yearned to feel the sunshine and rain on her skin on their daily strolls. Her solution was to harness Daphne to the wheelchair and train her to pull Jackie's chair. Her husband suggested that Jackie suspend a treat at the end a stick which Jackie could dangle just out of the reach of the great mutt. The 'donkey and carrot' trick worked perfectly and Jackie and Daphne took long strolls through the neighbourhood, although there were times when Jackie was irritated at how slow Daphne was at following commands.

One day when Jackie was particularly frustrated with Daphne, a man in a car stopped beside her and rolled down his window. Smiling at the two of them he said "What a beautiful dog you have there." Jackie turned to Daphne and grinned broadly. "Thank you," she said to the man. In her heart she said "Thank you God for reminding me to be grateful."

By the time Jackie attended a weekend retreat, she had done a lot of work on her spiritual path. It was inspiring to witness her gaining further insights during the weekend as she engaged deeply in each exercise. By Sunday morning, Jackie's small group drew in close, in rapt attention, as Jackie discussed her greatest fears.

"First I thought I was most afraid of dying. I spent a couple of years stuck on that thought. Eventually I realized I'm not actually that afraid of dying. I'm beginning to feel certain that when I die I will be fine." Her voice was low and calm.

"I also think maybe heaven is here and now, that we are creating it. This means I will stay here even after I die, but I'll be on a different wavelength. You can still see your family and you can still be there for them but they can't see you. So I told my kids if there is some way for me to comfort them or connect after I'm dead, I'm sure I'll be able to do it.

"I'm also exploring this idea that maybe you die when you've done what you needed to do. Maybe there are no early or accidental deaths. I have my human self and my spirit self. My human self will never be OK with dying – that's part of my humanity. But I also have a spirit, a soul. And, maybe all of our souls know exactly what's going on. So I now say to my kids 'Maybe your soul wanted to go down to earth and live with that family where the mom is going to die. Maybe you're supposed to experience that.'

"When I realized I wasn't afraid of dying, I thought maybe I'm afraid of my children suffering without me there to comfort them. But then I realized I'm not afraid of my children suffering. I've always been one of those moms who let them fall flat on their face. It doesn't bother me at all when they are wailing because their boyfriend broke up with them. I can listen to them and then I can leave it, because it's not my problem. I comfort them, but I don't try to remove things that are obstacles in their path.

"Maybe, suffering without me is part of what they have to do. That would be comforting, if I could believe that." Jackie's eyes moistened as she thought about her kids. The group was silent, waiting to hear what she would say next.

"For most of my life, I ignored the parts of myself I didn't like. I fought against the idea that I'm so emotional. Now I feel that 'I am wonderfully made' and so is everyone else. I don't want to spend time with my kids preparing them for my death anymore. I want to spend time showing them how wonderful they are. I've learned that my life is a lot better when I hold it with an open hand. Because I've been afraid, I've been holding on to my kids like this." Jackie lifts up her arm with a clenched fist. "But I will enjoy them much better if I hold them like this." She opens her hand, palm upward. "And that doesn't mean I don't love them. In fact, it is a blessed understanding of something larger than all of us."

Jackie finished her reflections about dying by telling the story about a little girl named Hope from her church who died of a brain tumor. Jackie's church choir had been invited to sing the song 'Morning has Broken' at the funeral and Jackie had agreed to sing a solo. Before the funeral the little girl's Godmother told the choir about the girl's life and explained the choice of the opening song.

The morning that Hope died, her mother held her in her arms and sang 'Morning has broken, like the first morning, black bird has spoken, like the first dawn'. They opened the window and on a sunny Thanksgiving Day Hope passed along.

Everyone in the choir was in tears when they heard the story. Jackie sang with the choir at the front of the church and she cried openly, visualizing Hope's mother singing the song to her on that last morning.

Before Jackie was to sing her solo, Father Jim gave the Homily which concluded with "Hope was beautiful and unique and we marvelled at her beauty, and then she was gone. This is what she had. This was her life. It was four years but it was complete."

Jackie stopped at this point in telling this story, the tears streaming down her face. "When Father Jim had finished his Homily something snapped in me. My fear of death started to melt away. I knew I was just like Hope. And that no matter how long I lived, my life would be complete."

Jackie finished her story, smiling through her tears. "I was a wreck after the Homily. I was crying so hard I couldn't even see the processional and I was thinking I wouldn't be able to sing my solo. So I prayed to myself 'Well God, I'm here. I'm either going to look like an idiot or not. It's going to be what it is.' And you know what? Somehow I did it. Afterwards people asked me how I could have sung so beautifully through all the tears. And I told them 'Well, I don't think it was me, actually.'

"My faith keeps getting stronger along the way. I make sure I leave space in my life for God to work. I spend more time with myself in meditation, doing yoga, and praying and less time worrying about getting everything done before I die. I tell myself each morning 'I will die when I am finished, when my life is complete.' I meander through my day letting the wind blow me where it will. It's quite a lovely existence."

CHAPTER 35

When Fear is the Teacher

From the perspective of many wisdom traditions, death is seen as the ultimate moment for the complete liberation of the mind from all entanglements, all sorrows, all separateness. If we look really deeply, we may see that suffering and freedom from suffering are embedded in each other. In the apparent darkness of death rests the light of freedom if only we can perceive it. Our practice and our very lives are also where we can see the light of this freedom.
Joan Halifax

Sunday morning. *From the first few words of Tim's lecture, people at the retreat straighten up and pay close attention. He delivers a spiritual message, illustrating that by embracing and working with our fears, we can heal our lives.*

We have already talked about how fear triggers the stress reaction and how you can learn to settle your physical reactions and your fearful thought patterns. The presence of fear, however, can also act as a catalyst for a whole new level of existential questioning and spiritual exploration.

Facing your fears can initiate a turning point in your life. The starting point is to look at fear directly. Often during the weekend retreats, people say their greatest fear is the unknown. They feel overwhelmed by the many unknowns on the cancer journey. They may ask themselves "Will I be cured? What happens if my cancer recurs? Will it grow quickly or spread to my vital organs? Will treatment be effective? How long will I live? How will my spouse or my kids cope if I die?"

As a young mother with a diagnosis of breast cancer put it, "Having a cancer diagnosis is like living in the land of the unknown."

People react in many different ways when facing the fear of the unknown. Some people try to stay positive or they bargain with God for a better outcome. Others obsess about worst case scenarios or become trapped in loops of despair or anger. Others may simply try to block out any awareness of their fear of looming unknowns. "I just don't go there!" declared one man with metastatic prostate cancer.

The fact is, though, even if everyone were to be cured of cancer, we would all still be living in the land of the unknown. We always have and always will. As much as we would like to control our health, or how long we live or the welfare of our loved ones, or anything else, the future is ultimately unknown.

The energy we use to avoid our fears or to try to banish them can actually feed them until those fears become bloated and exaggerated. Then our fears demand more energy to fight them back. Thus, a vicious cycle can emerge where the more we avoid our fears the more they grow and the more we struggle to avoid them.

Exploring our fear of the unknown might actually be helpful. On the one hand, thinking about fears can trigger more fear, and so we seem to feel better when we don't think about them at all. On the other hand, fear can also call us to investigate life more closely; to go beyond ourselves; to learn, to grow and to extend our selves beyond the limits of our comfort zone.

When I was a child I had terrible nightmares which lasted for many years. I would imagine that a 'boogey man' was perched in one corner of the room and that a 'swinging man' would crash through my window on the other side of the room. I spent the night looking back and forth, terrified that these two men would hold me down, and play scary movies in my head. I would also imagine there were monsters in the closet, snakes on the floor or that my bed was turning into a dragon. I would wake up screaming and crying.

My father would come and get into my bed to reassure me. After several years, when I was eight years old, he wanted to teach me to reassure myself so he quoted the famous line of Franklin Roosevelt: "There is nothing to fear but fear itself." That phrase blew my mind open. I began to repeat it over and over like a mantra to drive away the demons and to comfort myself. It was also like a Zen Koan, a type of Buddhist riddle, that pushed me beyond my normal way of thinking.

I have thought about and worked with fear ever since then. Even now, working as a psychotherapist, I realize that fear has a tendency to limit our horizons, to hold us back. When we are afraid, we shrink our world; we tend to stick with the known and stay away from the unknown. For instance, the people I counsel who are afraid of flying can't travel easily to Europe or the Caribbean. Some people who are scared of heights will not travel over the bridges that connect the twin cities where I live. They panic when they feel this vast sense of open space, and their fear prevents them from getting to the other side. In both cases, their phobias limit their ability to experience the world.

All of us are limited by fear in little ways every day. In social interactions, subtle forms of fear can keep us small and withdrawn. If we are scared of what people will think of us or if we are embarrassed to experience joy in simple interactions, we will keep ourselves within a narrow range of feelings and behaviours. We will 'play it safe', thereby limiting ourselves from the full potential of life.

The fear of intimacy is also a fear based in the unknown. You can ask yourself to what degree do you allow yourself to feel admiration or deep love for others, whether they are someone you have just met or someone you've known for a lifetime. If you are mindful, you can begin to see through the artificial boundaries that separate us as human beings and discover the intimacy that can crack your heart wide open. As you practice you can feel that tender heart-full connection with others more and more. You realize your love for others was always there - beneath the surface of distracting thoughts and fears.

However, we tend to protect ourselves from that degree of intimacy. We protect our hearts and stay within the known bounds of habitual interactions. We stay stuck, believing the maps in our minds of what we think we know about the other person. We may think 'I know this person, I know what their motives are. I know how they operate.' When we talk to ourselves that way we put a veil over our true perception and over the tenderness of our hearts.

We can approach our fears in a very different way by recognizing that every fear is actually a signal of being close to the threshold of psychological and spiritual growth. That's where we learn. That's where we can open our hearts to something new. It is like being able to fly to Mexico after overcoming the fear of flying. We can expand our horizons.

Instead of panicking when we feel anxious, we can try to stay relaxed, centered and mindful. We can ask ourselves: "What is this fear about in the larger journey of my life?" We might find that our fear is asking us to extend ourselves a little bit, just beyond the threshold of that particular fear. Every time we experience that little jolt of 'fight or flight', we can pay attention and say "Great! I know that there is a lesson for me here.

There's something I can learn from this experience. I can open up and actually extend myself into the realm of the unknown."

As we learn that fear is always workable, we can actually use the energy of our fear to overcome the fear itself. Remember what it is like to be a scared child standing at the edge of a diving board for the first time with all your friends shouting 'jump! Jump!' The adrenaline of being scared actually propelled you to jump, landing with a splash in the fresh water. In the same way, now as an adult, you can use this very energy of fear to initiate a similar jump into and beyond the fear.

The point is we don't need to get rid of our fear. We can learn to acknowledge our fears openly and honestly. We can talk about them with others and confront them directly in our own minds with moment-to-moment mindfulness.

When we pull a fear out of the darkened borders of our mind and openly face it, we begin to develop fearlessness, or a willingness to be *with* the fear and make friends with it. Practicing fearlessness doesn't mean that we will never have fear. It means that we can gradually learn to embrace the fear as an essential component of our life's journey. Feeling fear is feeling the energy of life itself.

We can learn to hold our fears like a mother holds a frightened child, with awareness and tenderness. Holding fear in this way allows us to use the energy of the fear to go forward. When we are totally honest with ourselves, we can find bravery within the experience of fear and embark on an adventure into the unknown.

The essence of spirituality, in some sense, is this process of embracing and staying with the unknown. The spiritual realm is bigger than ourselves and beyond what we can understand or control. Staying with an "I don't know" attitude as we experience our fear of the unknown is a spiritual practice that allows us to tap into something much bigger than our rational minds can conceive.

Fear of our Own Brilliance

Our fear of the unknown is not restricted just to the things that we think will hurt us or that we consider bad. We are equally afraid of our own brilliance. Part of what lies out there, in the land of the unknown, is our enlightened nature and our limitless potential – that tremendous energy and power that is our birthright. Nelson Mandella, the former president of South Africa, quoted Marianne Williamson in his inaugural speech:

"Our deepest fear is not that we are inadequate. Our deepest fear is that we are powerful beyond measure. It is our light, not our darkness that most frightens us. We ask ourselves: 'Who am I to be brilliant, gorgeous, talented, fabulous?' Actually, who are you *not* to be? You are a child of God. Your playing small does not serve the world. There is nothing enlightened about shrinking so that other people won't feel insecure around you. We are all meant to shine, as children do. We were born to make manifest the glory of God that is within us. It's not just in some of us; it's in everyone. And as we let our own light shine, we unconsciously give other people permission to do the same. As we are liberated from our own fear, our presence automatically liberates others."

We often hold ourselves back. We are afraid to acknowledge our brilliance and afraid to allow that divine being that we all are to shine through the usual mask we wear. This notion of manifesting 'the glory of God that is within us' scares us because it goes beyond our concept of comfortable world that we think we know. That vastness and power that we can tap into is definitely beyond anything that we can control. It is like a brilliant light that shines through us and can break us wide open.

It may seem paradoxical but contemplating death, the ultimate unknown, can open us up to the brilliance of life. We do know for certain that we will die but what lies behind that threshold is a great mystery. We may have a faith or we may speculate as to what happens after death, but the truth is we really don't know.

In many of the world's great spiritual traditions contemplating one's own mortality is a way of making contact with our spiritual essence here and now, a way to bring that energy into our life. When we deeply contemplate our mortality, or that of a loved one, we realize how every moment of life is totally unique, sacred and precious. This has been true in my own life.

The Story of My Dad

A number of years ago my mom gave me a call to say that my Dad had just come out of the shower and his face was drooping. He had a mini-stroke and was taken to the hospital. Within a week I flew out to visit them and see if I could be of service. By then he'd had a few more of these mini strokes. He seemed to be improving a little and was sent to rehab to learn to walk again.

He was doing okay but could barely speak. I remember helping him to go up some practice stairs. Although he was in rehabilitation, he was also in a place where he wasn't communicating the way he used to. He had been a great conversationalist who knew a little bit about everything. Now he was withdrawn and seemed lost.

He suffered another stroke and was sent back to the hospital. My brother and sister joined me and my Mom. At this point, my Dad was on a feeding tube because he couldn't swallow. The stroke had affected his ability to perceive his body in space and he had the sensation that he was being propelled through space at incredible speeds, feeling that he was about to crash into something.

He was trapped in a scary dream space, and now I was the one trying to comfort him during his nightmares. He was very strong and he would grip my hand very tightly and say "NO, NO, NO, NO, DON'T!" when he felt that he was about to crash. I spent my time at his side trying to comfort him.

As weeks passed, we recognized that things weren't going to get better. He was being kept alive by a feeding tube. We met with the doctors and the people from the hospice program. We thought about what he would have wanted in this situation. My father had lived a great life. He was almost 81 and he had been a successful businessman, very involved in his church, and a leader in the community. He loved skiing and hiking. In fact I had skied with him that January when he was 80 years old.

Eventually we decided to unplug the feeding tube and bring him home to die a natural death. My brother struggled with the decision. He is a philosopher and teaches ethics at the University of Colorado. I don't think he was comfortable with the idea of playing God, and he was working out all the philosophical ramifications in his mind. Mom was not really able to settle enough to touch the truth of the situation, that her husband was dying. She needed to be in a bit of denial at that time, which was totally natural. Nonetheless, we made the decision as a family to let him die.

On our way home, after making the decision at the hospital, my brother and I stopped to pick up some of his favourite Belgian beer. When we got home, my brother got out his guitar and started to play some of the songs that we used to sing with Dad around the campfire at our mountain camp. Tears started streaming down my cheeks. I thought about all those times, singing around the campfire, my Dad getting up early in the morning, catching trout and cooking them for breakfast. I felt this deep connection with my father, and I felt the terrible sense of loss. Looking at my brother who was gently crying as he played the guitar, I really took in that we were about to let my Dad die. As the great sense of loss began to flow through me, I just let myself sob and wail. It was very cathartic and healing for me to be fully present with my feelings.

Meanwhile, my Mom and my sister were in the kitchen, working on supper, and my Mom called out "Now Tim, you're the strong one. You're supposed to be the psychologist to help us through this." And I just wailed and cried some more. I let my feelings flow in full force. I couldn't stop at that point even if I wanted to. I did take to heart what she was saying and thought, "Yes, but this is the way I'm doing it, Mom. Let's feel this and really take it in and honour it for what it really is."

The next day, we brought Dad home. I rode in the ambulance with him, back to the house he had built when I was a child. We had a hospital bed brought in and we learned how to change the sheets and how to look after him.

I spent many hours just being at his side. We couldn't really have a conversation so I would meditate and try to join with him in the space where he was. He continued to live for twelve days. As time went by, we felt a sense of an inner radiance in the room. My Dad had been a very religious person so we recited the Lord's Prayer every day together, holding hands in a circle around him. We had the sense that he was there with us even though he could not respond.

I was on a late shift, starting at four in the morning, when I noticed his breathing start to change. He would take a full minute between breaths, then he would draw in another huge breath. I realized he would die soon so gathered my Mom, brother and sister. Then, right at dawn, as the sun was rising, he took his last breath. Peacefully he just moved on. It was very powerful for all of us to be there, to fully be there, united together, to honour the experience. I felt tremendous love for my brother, sister and Mom, tremendous admiration and respect. It bonded all of us together.

I share this experience to bring up and honour our mortality. I think it is an important part of a spiritual journey to make friends with death and to see death as an integral part of life's journey. In our society death is something that we tend to hide from. We don't want to think about it or talk about it. We try to sweep it under the rug. Whereas in other cultures, those based on the wisdom of contemplative practice, there are rituals and a process for embracing and celebrating the final transition of life.

This life is like a flash of lightning in the vastness of a cosmic eternity. When you are mindful of death and work with your fears, you begin to connect with how precious and sacred your life is in this very moment. You might then have a sense of the flash of this moment and this brief life as nested in the eternal, rather than being separate. You can see yourself in a larger context. You are more able to be both an individual and more than just an individual, at the same time. You are the sky out of which the flash of lightning comes.

Looking directly at and leaning into your fears awakens fearlessness. Bringing mindfulness and awareness directly into the experience of fear opens a welcoming doorway to the unknown – that vast realm of possibility and healing.

CHAPTER 36

Christine
Heal My Soul or Die Trying

Christine, a 40-year-old mother of two teenagers and former advertising executive, had a gut-wrenching decision to make. Her son was going to graduate from high school in four months and she was determined to be there, but the "miracle" drug she had been taking for two years for her blood cancer was no longer working. Her doctors told her the only remaining option was a bone marrow transplant but the chance of surviving this super high-dose chemotherapy was only 50 percent in the first hundred days. The alternative to a transplant was to go into palliative care and hope for yet another miracle drug to come along.

The following is an excerpt from a letter she sent to her CML (Chronic Myelogenous Leukemia) cancer support group explaining how she felt about her choices.

"I cannot see how this decision can be made in the rational realm. Each path requires embracing the unknowable, and trusting whatever happens. Each path is loaded with huge risks and lots of unknowns. Ultimately I am being asked to fully surrender to God/the Universe.

At my very core, I am vulnerable, fragile and somewhat powerless: fully human. I am also a Being unto myself and a part of a Greater Being: fully divine. My very existence is all the evidence I should require to see that I am worthy.

My journey began in unconsciousness. Now awareness grows bit by bit. It requires effort to grow towards wholeness and intimacy. I need to trust the Universe/God and myself to fulfill all my human needs, and the needs of my soul: harmony, sharing, and reverence for life. I have been working very hard to choose to live in love and trust—and I feel it's beginning to work."

Despite her spiritual approach, Christine continued to wrestle with this decision. When she sat down with her husband and kids around the kitchen table, she asked them if they thought she would walk away from the transplant alive. None of them raised their hands. They simply were not prepared to participate in her decision or face the reality of the situation. Christine desperately wanted to be alive for her kids but felt terribly alone.

She realized she needed to be by herself to make this decision; so in the deep cold of February, Christine went on a three-day solo retreat in a cottage on the shore of the Atlantic Ocean. When the owner of the cottage found out why Christine was in retreat, she gave Christine a set of Native Medicine Cards. Christine's spirits brightened as she viewed the medicine cards as a means of making her decision from an intuitive and spiritual realm. Derived from Native American spirituality, each card represents the spiritual and wisdom characteristics of a different animal totem. Shuffling and laying out the cards in formations can answer questions about different aspects of a situation.

Christine laid out seven cards in what is known as the 'totem spread'— one card for each of the four cardinal directions and one for above, below, and within. All the cards were insightful, but there were two which stood out as very significant for Christine.

The card in the east could be interpreted as her future, the direction of forward movement. Tears came to her eyes to see a Butterfly card in this position, for the butterfly represents transformation. Next, she contemplated her center card which represented her inner work. The hard-shelled Armadillo card in this position meant that she had to set strong boundaries, something she had been recently working on with her therapist. The Armadillo confirmed that not worrying about others' reactions was essential for her to trust her own intuition.

In a second reading, she laid the cards in a butterfly spread designed to bring insight at times of transition and to aid in decision making. She immediately noticed the Black Panther card, representing the power of embracing the unknown. This triggered in her a feeling of deep inner journey, connecting her to spiritual wisdom that lies beyond the self. At that moment, even though she was scared, Christine felt resolved not to undergo the transplant, and to embrace the unknown of no active treatment.

The months that followed were the darkest days in her life. Her body was deteriorating. She lay on her bed curled up in a fetal position, feeling lost and alone, bursting into sobs, thinking of her previous life. She had been a high powered professional with a successful marketing career, a loving mother and wife and an active community volunteer. Since she had been diagnosed with her leukemia, she had had to leave her work, and, with it, all it had meant to her self-esteem and a sense of structure in her life. She could no longer even make a simple nightly meal for her family. All this loss and her mounting fears snowballed into an avalanche of despair and darkness.

While floating in this abyss, Christine desperately wanted to feel connected to others, but instead she felt alone and disconnected. She had latched on to the idea of attending her son's graduation in four months, and then had bargained with God to attend her daughter's graduation four years later. But as Christine became weaker and weaker, the fear of dying swirled around in her mind.

Her doctors changed her medication again, with disastrous results. Her brain began to misfire and her mind went into a world of its own. Her daughter was terrified to find Christine at home babbling to herself. Fortunately, an elderly neighbour arrived and took Christine to the hospital, where she began to work with a wise psychiatrist.

In their first session, Christine shared her sense of having nothing left inside. She confided in the doctor that she didn't know whether she was going to live or die and it was too painful for her to be in that space. She wanted to redirect her time and energy, as she proclaimed, "to heal my soul or die trying." Her doctors found a drug that stabilized her cancer, and she was given a few more months to do her soul work.

Christine didn't know what healing her soul meant but understood that her fear was the leading edge of her personal and spiritual growth. She sought out a spiritual teacher, Alix, a wise woman trained in energy therapy. In one of their early sessions, Christine came in weeping and continued to cry uncontrollably. Alix, while attentive and present to her pain, realized Christine needed some energy work to ground her wild emotions and reconnect to her mind and to her body.

Alix told her, "You're like a drowning person out in the middle of the ocean with no one to save you. You need to stop flailing about. Calm yourself. Tread water as best as you can to preserve your energy for the work ahead. You have great inner resources and strength, now you need to find them." This was a turning point on Christine's spiritual journey. From this point on, she felt more secure in her own body, as if she had been thrown a lifesaver in the open waters.

In a later session, they spoke about Christine's persistent sense of unworthiness and her resistance to receiving love, nourishment and support from others. Christine reflected on her childhood. She had grown up as a French Catholic, and, as a child, felt a natural connection with a Divine Presence bigger than herself. She expressed this partially through innocent faith and obedience to the norms of family, school, and church.

As she entered adolescence, she began to explore a healthy rebellious side of her nature. In reaction to this, the nuns at her school were often cruel and uncompromising. Even though Christine understood from the stories of Christ that He loved and accepted everyone, the nuns didn't seem to accept her as she was. She felt the nuns instilled fear and guilt in the children to control their behaviour.

This harsh culture of guilt, and criticism, and feeling sinful as a child, led Christine to feel deeply unworthy. She would refer to the persistent negative voice inside her from the past as "Nunzilla." In her healing work with Alix, Christine found that much of her early conditioning from the nuns was still deeply embedded and affected how she lived her life—especially how she related to herself.

Her inner work began to take new spiritual directions. "I read many books that slowly initiated some major shifts in my inner landscape. I began to connect with myself and discovered value there after all. After a time, I managed to wrestle God away from Nunzilla, believing that surely God was greater than the 'Church God' of my youth. I am now relieved and inspired to discover God is greater than religion."

Working with Alix, Christine was able to integrate her emerging awareness with the pure spiritual understanding of her youth. She learned to use a simple prayer to stay connected with her own sacredness: "God spare me from the desire to seek love and approval. Allow me to know that abundant love and divine approval are already fully present right here, right now, and always."

Christine told Alix about a profound moment of opening and connection she experienced as a young mother. Holding her newborn son in her arms for the first time and gazing into his eyes, she felt transported into a different state. "I felt a deep sense of oneness with my baby and a union with everything in a flow of universal love. It was like a vast, pure realm of all potentiality. Then just as quickly as the understanding had come on, it faded, and I heard the sounds of nurses, other mothers in labour, and babies crying."

Alix asked Christine to put herself in the position of her son and to receive a mother's loving gaze pouring down on her, to be the baby and receive that vast love. This was a totally new experience for Christine and a wellspring of old tears burst forth. Christine realized that she was trying so hard 'to be strong' and 'to do it right'. All that effort, all that trying had become a kind of rigid armour that prevented love from getting in.

With this hint of a different way of being, Alix taught Christine to reconnect with the experience of receiving love by practicing this visualization in open-hearted meditation. Using the memory/image of a mother looking down on her child and the feeling of receiving love in her meditation, Christine began to gradually transform her underlying resistance to receiving love and support in her life.

Christine's second major issue was working with her fear of dying. While her doctors were keeping Christine alive with experimental therapies, she wavered between being energetic and being too tired to get off the couch. As part of her courageous approach of working with her fear, she asked her doctor to describe in detail what happens in a blast crisis, the fatal last phase of leukemia. She wanted to know what to expect, what it would feel like, and what kind of pain there would be.

"His description was ugly. I'm surprised he actually explained it to me, but I was desperate and told him I wouldn't leave the office unless he did. It's strange, but, since then, I don't plan for the future any more. I don't want to sound like I think that I am above all this, but I just decided at that time, 'Okay, I'm not planning for the future' – and I haven't."

Through the years of working with Alix, and in her own study and readings, Christine grappled deeply with her relationship with death. "It felt like Russian Roulette. There was a gun to my head and I thought, 'Well, what do you do with a gun to your head?' So I worked with that. I figured out how to ignore the gun, or just accept that the gun was always there. The biggest thing that was going to happen to me was that I was going to die. So how do I reframe that? I don't think about death as the ending point any more. I think of it as a transformation. I gave myself permission to believe that it is a transition point or change point, like when the caterpillar becomes the butterfly."

Christine doesn't hold too strongly to her beliefs about death though. "Once I let go of trying to know what was going to happen, I noticed that the real point is to live, and to experience life fully. I realized that to be open and available to whatever experience we have in the present was all we can do and all we need to do. I hadn't been open because I was bogged down with a million habitual patterns and conditioned thoughts and beliefs, and heaps of commonly held misconceptions.

Until I saw beyond these, I was not able to be present for the wonder and magic that is living.

"If there is no provable purpose, well then, let's make the purpose to live life fully. At least then, we all can love and be loved, and we can all do something beautiful with that. Worrying about dying became fruitless as far as I was concerned. It was an unnecessary worry, an unnecessary anxiety."

A few years later, when Christine continued to beat the odds with each successive therapy, her healer, Alix, was diagnosed with advanced ovarian cancer. Christine was deeply shocked. "It was one of those moments where the student becomes the teacher. All of a sudden, Alix was in this completely different space, and so was I. She was going to die and I was still living."

Christine grieved Alix's loss deeply but also took it as another profound teaching. Alix had helped Christine face her fear of death and then had demonstrated how to face it with dignity. Losing Alix opened Christine's soul to the realm of love and she knew that what she had learned from Alix, and their time together, could not possibly disappear from her heart.

It's been three years since that profound lesson. Sometimes living on the edge of death while looking fit and vibrant at other times, Christine has been deeply transformed. She now lives her life in three month segments, the interval between her bone marrow biopsies. For nine long years, the result of the biopsy has been the same - her leukemia has not responded to any treatment.

But on her twenty-seventh biopsy, Christine finally received fantastic news. Her cancer was going into remission. Only five percent of the cancer cells were left in her marrow and her prognosis was looking promising. Her brown eyes sparkled as she told this to everyone in the opening circle of our weekend retreat.

Remarkably, her attitude towards life did not change in any way with this great news. She was still living life to the fullest. During the weekend Christine was willing to cry openly, to laugh, to express her anger and to joke around. She even led a spontaneous round of the song *I can see clearly now the rain is gone* before we started one morning.

After the opening meditation on Sunday morning, she shared a dream she had the night before. "I was in what I guess was my house, but it didn't look like my house. There was an elephant in the basement. And the elephant was tired and wet and was having trouble walking. And so, finally, we let the elephant out and then it staggered outside and died. I was sad, but glad because it was tired and it was done. It was ready to let go."

Christine believes her 'elephant coming out of the basement to die in the open air' had something to do with letting go of old ways of thinking and the death of an inner belief system. She went on to explain "I made a conscious decision to heal my soul or die trying. A major part of this journey has been to explore what 'healing my soul' really means.

"My journey has been amazing in many ways. I wouldn't go back. I know some patients say, 'I wish I could just go back to my normal life.' But not for me. Holy mackerel, I don't want my old life back. I really, really like the way I am now, how I feel, and how I relate to others. It's unfortunate I had to go through it with a gun to my head, but I guess that is just the way that Spirit works.

"It's so easy to get distracted and discouraged, and get caught up in other illusions. We are often so busy looking for what we already have. It takes a lot of work though. This retreat has been a big reminder for me to stay on the path, to practice meditation every day, because it makes such a big difference when I do.

"I've learned that love is our default setting. We get in the way of ourselves sometimes, we get in the way of each other, and we get in the way of everything. When you cut all that out, then you can get back to see that love is everywhere, within and without, all around. Love and healing are everywhere and always available."

CHAPTER 37

The Story of My Grandmother

*The soul force is indestructible
and it goes on gaining power until
it transforms everyone it touches.*
Mohandas Ghandi

Sunday morning. *The people at the retreat get up slowly from yoga mats and sit back in their chairs. There is a deep calm on their faces; their eyes are open and receptive. Rob starts the talk on spirituality by telling a story about his grandmother.*

On the eve of my grandmother's 110th birthday, I got a call from her nursing home that she was having chest pain. I was worried she was having a heart attack and wouldn't make it to the big celebration that was being organized for the next day. That would be a shame because my grandmother was an amazing woman in many ways. She lived in her own apartment till 107, composed poetry up until her final months, and was an exceptional conversationalist with her many visitors. At 109, she pledged to herself that if she made 110, she'd dance on the table.

I rushed over to the Manor to see how sick she was. When I got to her floor I could hear the sounds of a lively violin coming from her room. Three of her great grandchildren, who are all excellent musicians, were serenading her with songs both lively and poignant.

Forgetting about the symptom of chest pains which had brought me there, I sat back and listened. The lyrics of one soft song started with 'the birds have flown away.' Listening to the beautiful harmony of their young voices I began to quietly cry realizing this would be one of the last memories I'd have of this extraordinary woman.

Grandma lay in her bed with a smile as broad as her face. As a doctor, I could tell that her body was very weak and she would not live much longer. But there she was, looking so happy, at peace, and absorbing every moment to the fullest. And more than that, there seemed to be a glow emanating from her that lit the room with warmth and joy.

I've experienced that same feeling at the bedside of many people who have released themselves into something so deep and mysterious that their inner light was obvious to everyone. Whenever this has happened, I have walked away from a simple conversation lighter on my feet and with a feeling that my heart had been stretched open.

My grandmother reminded me that a deep connection to spirit is possible even as the body is fading away and turning to dust. Over my years as a doctor, I've seen many of my patients who were able to let go into the spiritual realm, no longer identifying so closely with their bodies or even their personalities. Something like a pain crisis might dim their light, but once the pain was under control, and they could settle their minds, the brilliant light of their spirit could shine through again.

I remember a young mother I treated during her initial breast cancer diagnosis and again after it recurred. She had such exuberance for life regardless of her physical health. We had to delay her initial radiotherapy session because she had torn open her mastectomy sutures during a snowball fight with her kids.

Years later, when she was in the terminal phase of her life, I saw her again when she needed radiotherapy. Walking into her room, I could see that her body was frail, her skin yellow from cancer in the liver. But her face glowed and her eyes were filled with deep love. Though too weak to get up to greet me, she extended her arms up for a hug. Her voice rang out "Dr. Rutledge, I'm so happy to see you" as I leaned over for a long embrace.

She held not a hint of bitterness about her situation and I walked away from the clinic that afternoon with a lightness in my heart and an aspiration to share my love with others.

When we slow down, and are mindful of the true beauty of life, we can become more aware of the realm of spirit. It's here all the time, yet so obvious we can overlook it. I am truly grateful to my grandmother and so many of my patients who have lit the way, showing me the light of their living spirit even as their bodies were fading away.

P.S. As it turned out, my grandmother's chest pain resolved that night and, at the party next day, she conspired with two large men to place her wheelchair up on a large wooden table. She had everyone in attendance sing together songs to her like *I'm tired and I want to go home* — all the time her legs jigged and kicked in rhythm on the table.

CHAPTER 38

Circles Within Circles
Spirituality and Wholeness

When you surrender to what is, and so become
fully present, the past ceases to have any power.
The realm of being, which had been obscured
by the mind, then opens up. Suddenly a great
stillness arises within you, an unfathomable sense
of peace. And within that peace there is great joy,
and within that joy there is love, and at the inner
most core, there is the sacred, the immeasurable,
that which cannot be named.
Eckhart Tolle

Sunday morning. *Tim continues the talk about spirituality, offering insights from his diverse experience, and presenting a view that is accessible to people from all backgrounds.*

'The Ultimate Mystery' is a term that Father Thomas Keating, a contemplative teacher and author, has used to refer to the essential heart of spiritual life. The term hints at the fact that a spiritual life takes us beyond the known into the vastness of the unknown. Whatever form of spirituality we may practice, whether it is part of a faith-based community or a more secular approach, something deeply affirming and strangely inspirational happens when we allow ourselves to open to that realm that lies beyond our normal understanding. Witnessing the birth of a child or contemplating death and impermanence deeply can bring us to this state of awe and wonder, opening us to the palpable presence of something beyond ourselves.

The power of 'the Ultimate Mystery', or 'that which cannot be named', is that it is always fully present in our lives right here, right now. The spiritual journey is about learning to be open to and receive this presence into our lives by deliberately choosing to be conscious of it, even though it is beyond our normal understanding. For each of us to nurture our spiritual life, we must be willing to confront many paradoxes and embrace a lot of seeming confusion.

One of the paradoxes that we can embrace on the spiritual path is the paradox of unity and diversity. There are many ways to God, Spirit or 'the Ultimate Mystery', and at the same time, there is only one path: the path you are taking. Each of us has our own unique qualities as human beings and, at the same time, we all have access to something that unites us in a universal space beyond ourselves.

You can think of this wholeness in the experience of life as a big wagon wheel with the Ultimate Mystery at the center (see figure). All of the spokes that radiate towards the center are the different earthly ways of accessing the power of the Ultimate Mystery. In the very center, the complexity and diversity of the rims and spokes all come together into one point of simplicity and unity.

The many languages, cultures, religions and spiritual traditions of the world might be thought of as these different spokes that access the center.

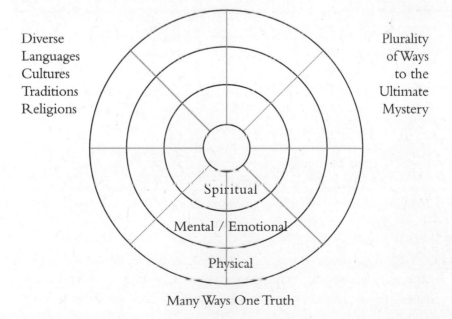

Diverse
Languages
Cultures
Traditions
Religions

Plurality
of Ways
to the
Ultimate
Mystery

Spiritual

Mental / Emotional

Physical

Many Ways One Truth

As well, in truth, each unique person actually has their own path and their own version of a spoke aligned with this universal point of unity. We all embody and participate in both the unity at the center and the diversity expressed throughout the wheel.

Thinking about this wagon wheel, we can say that the outer rim represents our life in the physical reality. This realm of physical reality is experienced by our senses and marked by impermanence. Everything changes here, nothing lasts. Time moves inextricably forward and all is subject to birth and death.

Moving inward toward the center, we pass into the mental/emotional realm which includes our emotions, language and storytelling, art and culture, the intellect and the realm of the mind. We often take this realm of our daily experience for granted, and yet it is in this realm we can transcend the inextricable march of time and remember our past and reflect on our plans for the future. We connect with the histories of our peoples and create visions for a better life for our children.

In indigenous cultures and in wisdom traditions around the world, the power of this mental/emotional realm is not taken for granted. Shamans, saints, and sages have referred to this realm as the dream-time, the dream-body, the soul, or the realm of visions and inspiration. In this realm, the boundaries between self and other are more fluid, and less rigid than in the physical world. For instance, as you read the stories of people who have transformed their cancer experience into a journey of the soul, you can probably identify with them to some degree, and feel their story mixing with your own.

Going beyond the realm of the mind and the richness of our collective imagination, and moving deeper toward the center point of the Ultimate Mystery, we come into a realm we might call the spiritual realm or spirit consciousness. In many traditions this is the realm of creation itself. Creation in this sense is not something that happened only once long ago but something that is always happening in the here and now. In this realm of spiritual consciousness the conventional concept of time is transcended to the extent that this very moment is synonymous with all eternity. There is only the now. This realization is what Eckhart Tolle calls *The Power of Now*.

With this spiritual consciousness all paradoxes begin to be resolved. Apparent opposites are brought together as two poles of one continuum. This is what is referred to in the language of mystical spirituality as 'nonduality' or 'not-two'. For example the earth's north and south poles are far apart yet they are still part of the one earth. All of the pairs of opposites from our normal ways of thinking such as inside and outside, subject and object, self and other, form and formless, heaven and earth, life and death, divinity and humanity are resolved into a kind of fluid oneness where apparent opposites are unified into one whole.

One way to open ourselves to the experience of this spiritual view is through meditation. For example, think of the opposites of inside and outside. Generally, we think there is an inside to ourselves and an outside. In meditation, when we pay close attention to the breath moving in and out, we begin to truly realize that there is a constant interchange between the atmosphere and our physical body. With mindfulness we realize that the same is true of drinking water and in assimilating the food we eat. Every part of our body is gradually being renewed and replenished in a constant open system of exchange with our physical environment. The concept of inside versus outside begins to evaporate.

Likewise in the realm of the mind or in the dream-time, we begin to notice that we cannot really claim sole ownership of our thoughts. For what would our thoughts consist of if there was not a constant interchange of information in the common forms of language we share? When you read the classics, for example, you are literally sharing in an exchange of information through the myths and stories of the evolving soul that go back thousands of years. Our thoughts can no longer be clearly categorized as our own or someone else's.

Experiencing Awareness Through Meditation

In meditation, when we are simply open and present, we can begin to connect with an experience of the space between our thoughts – the space of 'no thought' that is like the clear blue sky behind the clouds. As we become more accustomed to this experience, we can begin to note that there is a constant background to all of our diverse thoughts, emotions, and sensations of the physical body. Meditation, in this way, can help us to tune into the consistent presence of the Ultimate Mystery in our lives. Gradually we can come to experience the ultimate mystery vividly as a constant presence and the foundation of everything.

The great poet T.S. Eliot captures this beautifully:

At the still point of the turning world. Neither flesh nor fleshless;
Neither from nor towards; at the still point, there the dance is,
But neither arrest nor movement. And do not call it fixity,
Where past and future are gathered. Neither movement from nor towards,
Neither ascent nor decline. Except for the point, the still point,
There would be no dance, and there is only the dance.

The Value of Tuning in to the Realm of Spirituality on the Cancer Journey

Tuning in to the realm of spirituality can provide comfort and perspective even in the most troubling of times. As an analogy, imagine walking along a beach in the middle of a hurricane. The rain is pouring down in sheets as intense winds drive the water sidelong into your eyes and against your body and face. The winds rage in your ears as huge waves crash at your feet and threaten at any minute to wash you away. You are soaked to the bone and tossed and battered by the elements.

This same hurricane, viewed from a satellite twenty miles up in the sky, looks very different. From this aerial view it might seem like a beautiful blossoming rose of swirling cloud formations. Likewise, the same hurricane experienced from sixty feet below the water, where things are still and calm, seems only as a distant disturbance on the surface.

Learning to remember the spiritual perspective can give you a place of calm even in the midst of the storm. By cultivating a more spiritual perspective you can still appreciate the walk along the beach no matter what the weather.

We tend to see ourselves as existing only in a purely physical or materialistic version of reality. In other words, we tend to think of ourselves and experience ourselves as if we lived only on the very outer surface of the wagon wheel. This may seem to work for a while but often leads to a vague sense that there is something missing. We may experience a kind of restlessness and anxiety, or yearn for something more. We may try to appease this yearning through accumulating more things, more knowledge or more experiences. But, ultimately, none of these things are really satisfying. Our greatest yearning is to know deeper truths and to be more fully alive, genuine and whole.

Often times, a cancer diagnosis or another major crisis comes into our lives and forces us to grow beyond our old views. Our perspective can change in so many ways: to be mindful of the magic of life; to awaken to a way of being present to something that's greater than oneself; to know deeply that the Ultimate Mystery is already fully present no matter how your life unfolds. Whether we call it God, Goddess, Allah, Great Spirit, Basic Goodness, the Whole Universe, Cosmic Consciousness or the Creative Force doesn't really matter as much as learning how to experience the continuity of this presence in daily life.

In fact, the Ultimate Mystery is not far away or somewhere else. It is here, now. As Jesus said "The Kingdom of heaven is within and all around." It is only in our minds that we have created an alternative and false reality that this Ultimate Mystery is somewhere else. We are living in the dream of our own creation and that dream feels, in part, like a nightmare because it is not synchronized with the true majesty and splendour of the Ultimate Mystery.

Albert Einstein wrote "A human being is part of the whole, called by us 'universe'; a part limited in time and space. We experience ourselves, our thoughts and feelings as something separated from the rest – a kind of optical delusion of our consciousness. This delusion is a kind of prison for us, restricting us to our personal desires and to affection for a few persons nearest us. Our task must be to free ourselves from this prison by widening our circles of compassion to embrace all living creatures and the whole of Nature in its beauty."

From the perspective of the center of the wagon wheel's circle, we are the universe, one with the universal Ultimate Mystery, while, simultaneously, from the outer edges of the circle we are all independently existing beings living complex and diverse lives. We have our individual lives and individual consciousness, family life and family consciousness, community life and community consciousness, national life and national consciousness, world life and world consciousness, universal life and universal consciousness. These different aspects of who we are all occur simultaneously.

We frequently acknowledge this by saying our wholeness includes body, mind and spirit. Healing into wholeness, then, is learning to integrate the vastness of a spiritual perspective with the complexity of your personal mind and emotions. We draw on deep wisdom when we have insight from this bigger perspective that brings creativity and change into our lives.

This kind of wisdom can also have a profound effect on the well-being of our relationships and our physical health. If we really take this wholeness to heart in every moment of our lives, particularly while suffering, there is a quality of being with the suffering and being able to also hold a sense of spaciousness and openness in awareness around the suffering.

Many participants of weekend retreats have described this experience of holding their suffering and having a sense of peace at the same time. One elderly fellow with prostate cancer had travelled up to a weekend retreat by himself. His greatest worry was about the effect his cancer diagnosis had on his family. He was choked up with emotion as he grasped his hand against his heart, describing the gnawing pain he felt as he worried about his daughter. She had troubles with drug addiction and he worried that he wouldn't be there for her in the future. Through his tears, he also told the group that, amazingly, at the same time, he felt great joy, that life was carrying him along and things would work out somehow as they needed to, according to a plan more vast than his own.

Another women described her sorrow as she was grieving many losses in her life after her lymphoma recurred. The tears were welling up in her eyes, and then, in the same breath, she described how she also strangely felt a sense of bliss at times, as if she was being held by strong and loving arms when she needed it the most. She said that as she walks across what feels like a desert in her life, she feels as if there is a hand extended to her, helping her to steady her step and to offer her a drink of water.

Spirituality is such powerful medicine on a cancer journey or on any journey that includes suffering because it enables us to develop this sense of awareness to hold our suffering with loving tenderness even when we are hurting the most. We can regard our suffering with openness, acceptance and curiosity. We can learn to greet each experience as it arrives without judgment or aversion.

By cultivating this consciousness that is bigger than ourselves, we can actually celebrate experiences of all kinds. In the American schools of Japanese Zen, they call it 'Big Mind'. With Big Mind we can see the struggles and pain of the little 'me-mind' as if they were that hurricane disturbing the surface of the water. We can watch the disturbances attentively while also being one with the vast depths of peace and stillness below the surface, or being one with the vastness of sky above the hurricane, where the sun shines unobstructed by clouds.

Joining Heaven and Earth in the Goodness of the Human Heart

An ancient phrase proclaims, "All healing comes from heaven". Heaven, in the model of the big wagon wheel, is simply consciousness connected to the Ultimate Mystery. From this perspective, heaven is not far, far away or a place you can only go to in the afterlife. No, heaven in this sense is that Big Mind that connects us to a vastness beyond our personal selves and our struggles. It is a realm of tremendous clarity, creativity, and possibilities. It is the source of all, the ground of being. Our task is to join this heaven with earth which represents the practical details of our lives, including the health and well being of our physical bodies.

Bridging this vast heaven and our physical/earth experience is the energetic experience we call life. The stories of many people in this book demonstrate how, through facing their fears and coming to terms with distressing thoughts and difficult emotions, they transformed their life to view their cancer and everything else from a new perspective. When life is lived fully and consciously, embracing the energy of thoughts and emotions, then the wisdom from the realm of spirit or heaven is joined with our physical experience, earth.

Mindfulness practice, which gradually develops into Big Mind awareness in life, facilitates this transformation and healing. The energy of thoughts and emotions can be very tricky because, as Einstein says they can create, "a kind of optical delusion of our consciousness" when we regard ourselves as separate from others and the world around us. Mindfulness and awareness gradually reveal insight about interconnectedness and wholeness. Then through also cultivating loving kindness, compassion, and what we call heartfulness, we can begin to dispel this delusion of separateness, which Einstein says is like a prison. With loving-kindness, we learn to accept ourselves and others so we begin to feel more connected on our life journey, and then expanding beyond the small self, we can begin to truly relax. We say that heaven and earth join together in the goodness of the human heart.

And so we come to this understanding: the spiritual journey is one of opening your heart to love what is and to embrace each experience fully, without judgement, so that it can fully touch the tenderness of our good human heart. When we do this, we begin to draw on the healing power of heaven.

In the circle of healing, whether on a group retreat or in the privacy of one's own room reading this now, each of us can connect with our own heart energy and that of others. When the energy of the heart is shared, it blends and multiplies as it spreads around the circle. Respecting our differences, acknowledged on the outer rim of the circle, we also respect those aspects of life and spirit that are shared and universal.

As we gaze from the outer rim of our individuality in, toward the center of this circle, we become aware of an open space there. This open space we all share as a common ground of our being. This space represents the vast possibilities of change, healing and transformation. We can access wisdom, love and healing when we dip into the wellspring of this space. In the center of this common space, at the still point, life and death, arising and dissolving, are all one in the dance of the Ultimate Mystery.

CHAPTER 39

International Julie Day

"I'm not afraid of dying but I am afraid of not living"
Julie Easley

Julie grew up in the country surrounded by an extended family who loved each other and loved to celebrate. After graduating from university with a degree in anthropology, she moved away from home to what became an unhappy time in her life. She worked in a horrible job, skimping on the basic necessities to pay off a large student debt. Alone in her apartment, at age 23, Julie developed a cough, and soon found it difficult to swallow solid foods. A chest x-ray showed a mass the size of a grapefruit.

Julie instantly lost her illusion of being invincible and made a conscious effort to change her life. As a symbol to herself of the importance of self care, she went out and bought good underwear. With this shift came the feeling that her 'naïve' part of herself had died. She refers to life before cancer as BC, and after cancer as AD, as in After Death - death of her naïve self.

A biopsy confirmed Hodgkin's Lymphoma and Julie was slated for six cycles of chemotherapy and a month of radiation. Breaking this news to her family, on an Easter weekend, was heart-wrenching. At first she asked her mother to tell the other members of her family in another room because she couldn't bear seeing them break down. She caught her brother crying and felt guilty for making him feel so sad, but, in another sense, seeing her loved ones grieve gave her strength to show her family that she would be 'okay.' Her family pulled together and, in typical fashion, they danced and laughed and carried on like they always did.

During that weekend, Julie's uncle called to say Happy Easter to everyone. He himself had just been through cancer the year before. Julie walked to the bedroom for some privacy to talk to him on the phone. As she stepped through the doorway, it was like she was stepping over a line. Suddenly she was in his world and he was in hers. She knew what he felt and he knew what she felt, things no one else in the family could appreciate. They had a wonderful conversation and he was very supportive. Julie felt another shift, realized that she was changed forever, and that she was determined to 'get on the road.'

As a research nut, Julie knew every detail of the treatment that would ensue but her fears of chemotherapy were swirling in her mind. The night before the very first injection, Julie didn't sleep well, partly because the doctors had placed a needle in her chest they would later use to deliver the chemotherapy and she was worried it would fall out. In the middle of the night, she was awakened by a big storm. She thought, "Oh great, thunder and lightning, how much more miserable could this be? I'm going to go get chemo, I'm going to throw up, I'm going to lose my hair." A full symphony orchestra played a gloomy baroque piece in her head.

Then at six o'clock in the morning, a ray of light came through the window and shone directly on Julie's eyes. She woke up and stared straight into the light. In spite of her troubled night, something shifted subconsciously and she knew she was going to be okay.

Walking into the oncology unit for the first time, she burst into tears. "I felt like I was walking to the lethal injection chamber. I felt like I was on death row. How symbolic is that? It was the death of another part of me. But this was going to save my life, not kill me." At the same time as experiencing these fears, she felt like a butterfly emerging from her cocoon.

On May 11, her first day of chemotherapy, the first leaf of spring appeared on the maple tree outside of her bedroom window. Julie chooses to celebrate this first day of chemo even though she wavered between a deep sense of peace and being terrified of side effects. A new phase in her life had begun.

The chemotherapy was given every two weeks for six months. The first week of each cycle made her feel like 'crap' and the second week was a 'better version of crap.' By the fourteenth day, the day before her next cycle, she was well enough to eat whatever she wanted. Greek Salad. French fries. Anything. Everything. Julie's family called it 'Chemo Eve' and they decided to celebrate. "We'd always been about celebrating everything. We laugh hard and we cry hard. We're really about acknowledging the good, but it was an effort to learn to celebrate in the face of adversity."

Chemo Eve prompted poems like 'It was the night before Chemo and all through the house' Julie's brother, a professional musician, wrote other Chemo songs like 'On the first day of Chemo, my true love gave to me…' They had a party every two weeks and the word spread to other family and friends. On one Chemo Eve, Julie's Grade 2 teacher, who hadn't seen Julie in over ten years, travelled to their country home to organize 'Mexican Night.' On another Chemo Eve, Julie's crazy cousins cut down a huge evergreen. They set it in the kitchen and decorated it with syringes, hats, cans of supplement and rubber gloves.

Hosting Chemo Eve not only became a diversion but a warm show of support. Julie learned that her family and friends needed to feel needed – to be able to do something. Not only did Julie feel better after each Chemo Eve, even when she was exhausted, but her family and friends felt better too.

Chemotherapy was not easy even with all this love holding her up. On the first day of each cycle, Julie would vomit in the parking lot in anticipation of the chemotherapy. Suddenly the hospital smelt like 'they cleaned the place with urine.' Julie gained a huge appreciation for people challenged by mental issues because she understood the cause of her anticipatory nausea was psychological and there was nothing she could do about it.

At the halfway point of the chemotherapy, when everyone tried to encourage her saying the glass was 'half full', Julie felt terrible. September was always a time of new beginnings and she was trapped in bed. She decided she needed to learn how to be sick. She needed to learn to stop living in the future and just be with the present. While her friends were out camping, she set up her mattress in a tent in the kitchen.

On the last day of chemo she hugged her nurses good-bye. She put on her new tap shoes (a Chemo Eve present) and literally danced her way out of the clinic. "It was a pretty poor sight considering I don't know how to tap dance, but it was symbolic for me. I walked out of there with my head up. Cancer was not going to get me. I had made it through the worst time of my life."

Nonetheless, Julie bawled her eyes out in the parking lot, tears of exhaustion. The last leaf had fallen off the maple tree outside her window.

A month later on Christmas Eve, having finished the last of her radiotherapy treatments, Julie's emotions came down from her upper level of coping. Even though she got her period and eyebrows for Christmas, which was exciting to her, she felt guilty and questioned why she was not ecstatic? "This was the time I should be celebrating. But it was a scary place to be."

Julie was having an identity crisis. "It felt like someone handed me the rest of my life back and said 'There, go on your way.' Well, what do I do with this? Who am I? What am I? I had been 'Julie with the curly brown hair'. I did this. I did that. That's who I was and now I am 'Julie who had cancer'. That was my new identity. But now I'm finished treatment and am supposed to be on my merry way? I felt confused. That's when I broke down."

Julie went into a depression and decided to see a therapist. She cried continuously for a week, but not about cancer. It was about what kind of job she could get because she was asking herself what she was going to do after cancer that would ever have any real meaning. Julie's Mom took her to a guidance counsellor.

"Poor little, bald, skinny thing that I was, I crawled out of bed to go to a career counsellor. It was the best thing. She said to me, 'Where's your passion? What is it you want out of life?' She meant it career wise, but I heard it on such a higher level: 'What is my passion? Who am I? What is it that makes me, me?' I had to fight my way out of this depression, acknowledge it, embrace it, let myself cry. And then I said 'okay, what am I going to do about it?'"

In the cold of January, with nine dollars in her bank account, a $26,000 drug bill, and no health insurance, Julie needed time to learn how to be well again. By advocating for herself, she was granted social assistance for six months which meant her drug bill was paid for by the government. At first she struggled with the guilt of not working but soon realized the task of healing would take her full attention.

Alone in the house, still weakened from chemo, she chose to set small goals for herself and not look too far ahead. She bought a soup cookbook and made soup each day. This simple task changed her life. Julie learned to nurture herself in a simple and profound way.

Spending time alone, Julie started to feel the weight of what had happened. She'd ask herself "Did I dream this?" and then feel some sense of panic. She would have to consciously remember to breathe. She practiced breathing in the positive and blowing out the negative. She'd breathe in the positive, whether it was the smell of the soup or even the air, and, on the out-breath, she'd actually visualize the negative thoughts blowing out of her mouth. She started this ritual for herself and, to this day, uses this coping mechanism whenever she feels overwhelmed.

As part of reviewing her whole experience, Julie realized that she needed to give herself a break. "I just went through cancer. Of course I'm going to feel this way. I started acknowledging it was okay to feel the negative emotions. This is what people feel like.

"I had to learn to be consciously aware of my own emotional wellness. I felt like I was disconnected, that my physical body had somehow been separated from my mind. Yet through cancer, and especially when I had the anticipatory nausea, I had learned that my mind and body are so very connected. I had to connect my mind to my body in a positive way, to put the pieces back together."

Julie still had to figure out what she wanted to do for work. Through these tumultuous few months, she realized the cancer diagnosis may have provided her with a purpose. Julie had an interest in medical anthropology and she happened to find a professor who was looking for a research assistant for a research study on the perceptions of cancer and health seeking behaviour. Julie was accepted into a PhD program in medical anthropology and she has worked hard ever since studying the effects of cancer on the lives of young adults.

Along with her determination to make a difference in the world, she expresses a 'joie de vivre' in every aspect of her life. Her appreciation for living peaks each year on May 11, the anniversary of her first day of chemotherapy. For Julie and many of her friends and family, May 11 is 'International Julie Day'. On that day she doesn't want to receive gifts. Instead she wants her family and friends to take some time to reflect on life and to do something loving for themselves.

For Julie, no matter what is happening in her work world, she will take 'International Julie Day' off to do something special for herself. She may go to the spa for a facial or buy a CD of her favourite music. "It's like laughing in the face of cancer. I choose to celebrate. You can't take that away from me."

Every year, she also writes a letter to herself. She chooses to go back and acknowledge the journey that has made her who she is today. She firmly believes that the strength that she has now is largely because of cancer. Every May 11, Julie will walk quietly through the woods and look at the leaves on the maples that are beginning to bud again.

CHAPTER 40

"Julie, meet Randy"

Eighteen months since completing her chemotherapy, Julie, age 25, sits in the library contemplating her life. She's researching how cancer affects the lives of young adults like herself. She is grateful to have found her vocation out of the angst and inspiration of her cancer journey. But she also knows life is for the living – to laugh, to cry, to dance and to dream. This particular afternoon, she decides to see her favourite local band play in the university pub.

At 29, Randy was a vibrant and outgoing musician who was loved by many when he began to lose weight and suffer from stomach cramps. Surgeons opened his belly to discover that a rare and aggressive form of colon cancer had spread throughout his abdominal cavity and to his liver. They quickly closed him up and told his family there was nothing they could do, and that he may have only a week to live – at most three months.

Randy had different plans. The handsome young man was determined to live but felt self-conscious with a colostomy bag and a tube in his side to drain his urine. He lamented to his mother "How could anyone ever love me when I can't even love myself this way?" Three months to the day after his operation, on the day his doctors expected him to be dead, Randy finally mustered the courage to go out for the first time. He wanted to see his close friend, Tom, who was playing in a band that afternoon.

Julie walked in the backdoor of the pub while Randy entered in the front. Julie went to chat with the band members between sets. Tom, one of the band members, looked sad and told Julie he had recently found out that a close friend had terminal colon cancer. As they were chatting, Tom looked up and was surprised to see Randy and said "Oh my God, here he is now. Julie, meet Randy."

The instant their eyes met, Julie recognized something of herself in Randy – there was a searching in his eyes and a longing for something that was so familiar to her. They were in the same world, a place that those without a cancer diagnosis can't fully understand. The noise of the pub seemed to fall away as they shared their stories. Julie volunteered to do a literature search to help 'save Randy's life.' They exchanged email addresses. Randy went home and told his Mom that he had met an angel.

Because Julie worked in the hospital, she could easily pop down to see Randy whenever he was on chemo. She remembered, from when she had chemo, that having someone just sit with her was comforting. And so she sat with Randy.

Julie and Randy talked about everything. Julie reflects: "I wasn't afraid to go to the depths of the horrible with him – and come back up. And I think for him it was an outlet – he didn't have to protect me like he protected his family.

"I would mean to stop by for five minutes and I'd end up staying for four hours. He was so captivating to talk to. We laughed and laughed. Friends would be lined up down the hallway. He was so funny. He always had something to say. So I became obsessed. I couldn't wait to go down after work to have a laugh or share a story."

One night, when she found out no one was staying with Randy, Julie offered to spend the night in his hospital room. She knew Randy didn't like to spend the night alone because it was really hard for him to get up and move around.

People didn't understand why Julie, a beautiful young woman, would choose to fall in love with a man with a terminal illness. Julie found it frustrating to justify something that was just so natural to her. She felt she didn't have any control over it. "It was Randy. He was a beautiful person with whom I had an amazing connection right off the bat. People would say 'Think about you. You're getting too emotionally attached. This is going to be hard on you if something happens. What if this? What if that?' It was constant.

"Even the nurses would come in and say 'What about you?' But it wasn't about me. It was about us. Let's just take every day and every minute for what it is. Maybe this was something I learned from having cancer myself. That experience changed me as an individual. I don't look too far ahead. Yes, I have long term goals. But I've learned to take everything for what it is right now.

"Randy's health wavered. Five times he was told he'd be dead within the week. He was so full of life despite fighting for every scrap of it. That's probably why I fell in love with him. What I learned from him, from day one, was the strength of the human spirit. At one point he threw up buckets every hour on the hour. It was just unbelievable circumstances, and yet every morning he got up with a smile, and laughed and made a joke with the nurses."

In the cold of February, with a huge winter snow storm about to hit the region, Randy was accidentally given a near-lethal dose of morphine. He was revived in time but forced to stay awake for hours afterwards, making sure he wouldn't lapse into a coma and die. A large syringe of the antidote to morphine was taped to the wall above his bed, an image that continued to haunt him.

Even after he was safely through this spell, Randy wouldn't allow himself to fall asleep for fear of dying. Julie sat at his bedside, also worried if he'd make it through the night, watching his every breath. Finally Randy invited Julie into his bed. Julie wrapped her arms around him, placing her hand over his heart, feeling his every breath. She would know he was OK, and he would know that she knew. With this comfort it was like the peace of the world came over both of them and they fell asleep immediately. It snowed over four feet during the storm. With no visitors for two days, Julie held onto Randy in a deep and healing sleep.

Then Julie basically moved into the hospital with him. It felt like they were living in their own apartment. They had a little kitchenette and a little living room section where Randy had his chair. He had his home office where he had his recording equipment in the corner. And they had the hospital bed. In the reflection from the TV screen they could almost see a hallway down to the rest of their 'house'. Making up detailed descriptions of what was down the hallway became an evening pastime. It was magical for Julie to be able to share her craziest dreams and have someone to run with them even though they were in such a confined space.

Unfortunately, Randy's tumors were slowly progressing. The hospital staff tried to put him in Palliative Care, but he refused. One day, Randy's doctor ran into a group of Randy's family and friends just outside Randy's door. The doctor told everyone that Randy had very little time left.

Saddened by this news, the group walked into Randy's room only to find Randy out of bed for the first time in several days, standing with guitar in hand, composing a song. He had decided that he was going to record his solo CD, a project that would take several weeks for him and his musician friends to complete.

Randy's strength began to return. The experimental chemotherapy seemed to be working. His nausea got better. He started to eat and returned home. Julie remembers clearly. "We were given this miracle week. It was a gift. He felt like getting out of bed and we even had a day when we could go to the park. We walked around for an hour and a half."

Randy had something special for Julie – a ring he was given when he was a baby with a little letter 'R' inscribed on it. "He gave me this ring in a very sweet and quiet way. He gave it to me as a thank you but also with true love."

But the miracle week came to a crashing halt. The next morning Randy had a seizure and was rushed to the emergency room in a coma. The doctors there didn't think he would live long enough to reach the intensive care unit. A blood clot had broken off and lodged in his lung. His heart was labouring to overcome the blockage.

Julie rushed in from work. Randy woke up just in time to see her coming in. He winked and smiled at her. But the doctors could see that his organs were failing. Despite their pleas to have him agree to a 'do not resuscitate' order, Randy refused. He told them if he was going down, he would go down fighting. But on some level he knew he was dying and he wanted to say goodbye to his family and friends.

Randy held on, hour after hour. His Dad flew in by plane. Musician friends were tracked down at a distant music festival. Everyone arrived in time.

Randy greeted each one with a joke and a hug even as his body was weakening. Julie sang to him to pass the time.

Another blood clot travelled to his lungs and his breathing became more laboured. Finally, a nurse convinced Randy that, if he died, resuscitation would be both barbaric and pointless. Randy finally conceded. "OK then. Just let me go." Then his next words were "Can I have a Coke?" Everyone laughed and he savoured his last drink.

One by one, everyone said their goodbyes. His Mother leaned over her dying son. He reached up and hugged her ."I love you, mom."

With tears streaming down their cheeks, Randy's loved ones were gathered and holding hands in a circle around the bed, each echoing "I love you" in their own way.

Randy looked up to Julie "Can you hop in here?", asking her to join him in the bed. Julie tried to put her arms around him as she always had but Randy insisted on wrapping his arms around her. Julie gave in, letting herself be held in a profound love. The last thing he said was "I'm glad you're here", and then he closed his eyes and passed on.

Julie reflected later on the whole experience: "Not only do I not fear death, after having witnessed it, but I realized it was truly beautiful.

"It was really sad though, but if there's any consolation, it's this: if there was a way to go, that would be the way I would want to go. I'd want the person I love in bed beside me surrounded by my family hearing those loving words.

"Randy and I didn't have a past together, and sadly we didn't have a future either – we only had the present. And we managed to live every minute of it together, to the absolute fullest despite the circumstances. It is a lesson I carry forward: to enjoy every day for what it is in that moment.

"Who knows what the future holds for me. But to have known that depth of love is all I need. It existed for me. In such a short period of time, Randy gave me the most amazing memories. He gave me a journey, for myself and for us together. That's something I'll never forget."

CHAPTER 41

Closing Circle

The day will come when,
after harnessing the winds,
the tides, and gravitation,
we shall harness the energies of love.
And on that day,
for the second time in the history of the world,
we will have discovered fire.
Teilhard de Chardin

Sunday afternoon. *A bubbling energy fills the air as people begin to assemble into a healing circle. Some initially cluster in small groups, talking seriously or laughing and having fun. A few take to their chairs quickly, happy to rest and reflect on what has been an intense weekend.*

This group of fifty arrived on Friday night as strangers, nervous and excited. Now, two days later, after eating lunch in this healing community, their faces have softened and their eyes radiate a subtle sense of peace and joy. Along with this buoyant and loving energy, though, is an underlying sense of sadness. This is the last exercise of the weekend and they're soon to say goodbye.

Tim begins with a meditation, bringing the group back into a focused and grounded state. He has them mentally review their experience, from the time of their first intention to attend the retreat, to arriving on Friday evening to this large circle of chairs and participating in the various exercises and discussions throughout the weekend. His meditation instruction concludes with a loving-kindness visualization:

Reconnect with your heart
Remembering that it is always available
The universal quality of loving kindness is bigger than us but we are also part of it
Feel your heart opening and warming as if it were the radiant sun

Extend that sunlight from your heart outward so every cell of your body is drenched in that light
And all of your emotions and thoughts and the comings and goings of everyday concerns are held in the light of loving kindness
This love can extend beyond yourself
Feel that radiant light, that connection to every other heart
To your loved ones and friends and beyond to everyone everywhere
Review the weekend [and this book] in your mind in your own way
Look for those little moments, the little light bulbs in your head that allowed you to step outside the old ways of seeing things and begin to contemplate new possibilities
Contemplate your own unique insights, your own perspective and what you want to take home with you and how you want to go forward from this day onward.

Rob then instructs everyone to write down on a small card one or two of the insights they gained from the weekend. Some people begin to scribble their thoughts and reflections. Others stare into space for a few moments, distilling their insights to three or four words. A few will compose a poem or remember a famous quote. In turn, they will share with the large group what they have written.

Rob asks for a volunteer to begin. Gone is the awkward silence from Friday night's opening circle. There's a quiet buzz as they smile or wink at each other from across the circle.

Leon takes the microphone first. An immediate stillness fills the room. This brave young man with the bald head and a swollen eyelid has a softness and yet such a strong and reassuring presence. His quiet confidence speaks of a deep connection to spirit. Our hearts expand in rawness, admiration, and anticipation.

On Friday night Leon's wife, Suzie, was first to introduce him. They sat across from each other in the large circle, arriving late and taking the last two available chairs. With her first few words "I don't have cancer; my husband does," she began to cry. Leon walked across the circle to sit at his wife's feet. His presence was calming as he held her hand and smiled lovingly up at her.

Six years ago Leon was diagnosed with what was thought to be a highly curable testicular cancer when he was serving overseas in the military. In the week between his diagnosis and starting high-dose chemotherapy, he and Suzie conceived their first child. Two years ago his cancer recurred in the lung and liver and he went through a stem-cell transplant. Their second child was conceived at that time despite Leon being told that he was infertile. Finding out his tumor has recurred again, Leon sees his two young boys as his source of strength. He will fight for every extra day to be with them.

Now on Sunday afternoon, Leon looks relaxed sitting beside his wife. He smiles broadly and reads the card that summarizes his insight gained on the weekend. "Suzie wrote this down for me because my hand isn't working now. I summed it up like this: I'm being taken care of even when I feel I'm alone.

"It reminds me of a religious figurine a friend gave me. The story called 'Footsteps in the Sand' is written on it." Leon gives a shortened version of the classic fable. "A gentleman is walking in a desert and the Lord is beside him. The Lord tells him that He will always be with him. In his darkest hour, the man notices only a single set of footprints in the sand. So he asks the Lord, 'Why did you leave me in my darkest hour?' The Lord replies, "I never left you. I carried you. That's why there was only the single set of footprints."

Leon pauses and reflects on what this means for his life, "Even when I don't realize I'm being taken care of, there's always someone or something there beside me. That's the biggest thing I take away from this weekend." As he hands over the microphone, he puts his arm around Suzie's shoulder.

Suzie has been transformed this weekend. In recent months, she has been reluctant to talk about the "elephant in the middle of the room" but on Friday night, when they got home, Leon talked directly about making sure their financial affairs were in order. Suzie was saddened by the discussion but also inspired by Leon's resolve to take care of his family. She has spoken openly in her small groups with warmth and intelligence. She has let out many tears over the past two days and now addresses the group.

"I didn't know what to expect this weekend. My mother encouraged me to come. She does visualization and shares her experiences with me—they're really vivid. But I just thought it was a bit crazy." Suzie stops and laughs along with the group. "And now I understand how powerful they can be. Things come into your life when you need them. And I guess this is the time." Her voice becomes thin and her eyes moisten.

"I realized from this weekend that I'm a very emotional person but I've suppressed it for a long time, especially since Leon got sick. I don't like being emotional because I feel really vulnerable, like I'm out of control.

But that's the truth—I am out of control, at least for some things. And I didn't realize what was going on with me. The weekend taught me that if I don't look after myself I can't look after anybody else.

"The other thing is Leon and I have a really open relationship. But in the last few months we stopped talking about the things that were bothering us. It was like we were taking a break from all the bad news but we felt like there was nothing left to talk about.

"We have a happy home environment for the kids. There's lots of positive energy in the house but lately it didn't feel real." Suzie is on the verge of tears again. Leon has one arm over her back and with his other hand he offers her a tissue. The power of his gaze wraps Suzie in a blanket of loving kindness. His are the footprints that mark the path as he carries her through the desert.

Suzie smiles at her husband and continues with a strong voice. "But last night, sitting around with Grandma and the kids—I felt the joy again. I let the kids stay up late and read bedtime stories to them. I just loved it. We were back to where we used to be. Back to being happy and just experiencing it."

Leon looks at his wife with eyes radiating deep compassion and caring. Suzie is being imprinted with a love that will never leave her.

When Suzie passes the microphone along, I realize I've forgotten to tell people to put the cards they are holding into a wooden bowl that will be passed along with the microphone. I admit my mistake to the group and add in a mocking tone, "…but I still love myself." The group is quick to laugh and will continue to tease me and joke with each other between sharing their insights.

Alison, a woman in her late forties, who has been treated successfully for early breast cancer, lets the laughter subside. She begins by identifying the feeling she is experiencing here in the closing circle, something that so many other people have tried to describe over the years. "We humans all yearn to be compassionate and loving but we don't always find the situation to express that." She pauses and reflects "When I'm at the grocery store I don't normally express loving kindness. This weekend has provided the perfect opportunity."

Beside her sits Pam, a 60-year-old woman with advanced lung cancer. She and Alison were strangers who shared the four-hour drive from another city to the retreat and now seem like life-long friends. Pam has struggled in her relationships "to be taken seriously," especially when discussing complementary therapy with her oncologist. Pam also focuses on this new-found dimension. "During this weekend I found the inner power and the inner love to connect with strangers."

Many others described this mysterious love and connection, this magical web of humanity, this "weaving in and out of intertwining spirits." By joining in the healing circle, a light of love shines so brightly that at some point it seems as if the space between people in the circle literally becomes sparkling with love. This sensation of healing light begins with lines of connection joining one heart to another heart across the circle; then at some point the light catches fire and shows the unique glow around and within each person. Each person in the circle will walk away knowing, some for the first time in their lives, that love and deep human caring is possible in their lives.

Rick has this glow as he rubs his wife's back and listens intently to each person's reflection. He is in the midst of hormone and radiation treatment for an advanced but potentially curable prostate cancer. He drives a truck for the postal service and races cars as a hobby. He has also been touched by "a bond amongst all of us that I would never have thought was possible." He says this has opened him up to an emotion he didn't know he had and that it can help him grow.

Rick continues with his insight. "Most of us seem to be afraid of the unknown. We don't know about tomorrow or the next day. We can't predict what the future will bring. Through facing that fear, I have come to the conclusion that the future is right now.

"We need to take the time to enjoy the beautiful world out there and to live for right now. This morning when my wife and I were getting in the car to come here, we were running late as always. I was walking out into the front yard and there were these yellow daffodils just starting to unfold from their green stems. You can just see the little flower beginning to poke through. Then in my head there are the two voices.

"The first voice said, 'Ah, look at the beautiful daffodils.' "The second voice said, 'No, there is no time. We've got to go. We're late.' "Then the first voice said, 'No, look at the daffodils.'"

Rick adds "I can't say I've really looked at daffodils before. I really like working in the yard but I don't usually dwell on whether the daffodils are growing or not.

"On your way out this afternoon, stop and look at the beautiful plum trees. Stop and smell them; they are absolutely wonderful. Maybe that's the purpose of us having our struggles with our health and with staring death in the face. We learn to enjoy our lives more than we did before, to really take the time to acknowledge how beautiful life can be."

The next woman to take the microphone has a gravelly voice. "I can now say the word cancer." Another woman who looked so tense on Friday night, after practicing the loving kindness meditation, says that she can slow down now. "I can now be soft. I don't have to be strong all the time."

A woman who is coming to accept her self-image after a double mastectomy quotes Psalm 1:39: "God looks at us as a whole person."

Shannon, a young woman with breast cancer who has taken her healing journey very seriously concludes with the image of "jumping off the high diving board of fear—and landing with a cleansing splash in the pool of strength, courage, love and mindfulness."

Caroline is a beautiful actress who left a successful career in the city to return home to help her mother recover from breast cancer chemotherapy. "I moved back home to be near my family and have a sense of community." Her voice breaks and she's almost crying and smiling at the same time. "This weekend reminded me that in some cultures, when the men go off to war and then come back, the whole village will actually mourn and wail and cry. They will help the warriors heal, because the warriors have had to kill and do things they didn't like. So the community would take on that pain and sorrow. Everyone would feel the pain to help the healing."

She adds, "This weekend wasn't about cancer. It was about the power of the human spirit. Nothing can hold back the power of truth, pain, and the lightness of being."

Sandra, Caroline's mother, has wiped a few tears away as she takes the microphone from her daughter. She fakes a hillbilly accent and says "That's my girl." With the group laughing along, she points to the hotel conference room. "I almost feel this weekend we've spent on an island, it's called Survivor Delta Hotel, but nobody is getting voted off."

Sandra continues seriously, "Cancer has taught me a lot about living. It's a gift wrapped in duct tape. You have to pull at it a lot to get down to where it's good." Many people chuckle at the image but they see the wisdom in these words.

Sandra finishes with a poem she has just written:

Fears exposed for what they are
Disasters waiting to occur
Dissipated into air
Blasted out by loving care.
Be not afraid.

The group nods in gratitude and then continues. Silence. Contemplation. Laughter. More reflections and insights. Intensity and release. The group is breathing in and out as one body in the universal cycles of contraction and expansion.

The next to speak is a large woman who has also written a poem. She has acted as a small group facilitator during the weekend, having herself been treated for breast cancer years ago. She says "From the weekend I realized I need to give myself a hug every day. You know we're so good at sharing our love and giving our love to others, but loving ourselves and loving our body is a chore sometimes. I wrote down "I need to love my body— my own body." She adds that 'body' could also be understood as the community of people in our lives.

She then reads a poem she wrote moments before which she calls "Body Whispers":

Be gentle with me,
Be kind to me,
Remember to love me,
Take care of me,
So I can carry you through the life that comes to you.

There is a short silence as the simple beauty of this poem sinks in, then a spontaneous swell of applause.

The next lady is very spry for her 75 years. She takes the microphone and pretends to be irritated by this poem. "You said what I was going to say," she says, and throws her card in the wooden bowl and pretends she's finished. The group laughs again, enjoying her little comedy act and the released tension. They'll continue to ride these waves of emotion and insight. The energy in the room rises and falls like ocean swells.

Another woman follows, saying she was transformed by the bowl of loving kindness meditation. "I am going home with this big bowl of feelings. I have learned that it is best to recognize my stress and fears and those things that give me pain. I have learned that I can take them like putting together flour and vanilla for a cake. I can put them in my big bowl and I can fill that bowl with light and energy and can stir it all up. Then, with the light and energy, all the bad things I've acknowledged can make a good cake. I don't have to hide them back up in my cupboard somewhere. No, I can take that cake of light and energy and put it back into my heart."

The circle is drawing to a close. The last reflection comes from a woman whose husband has incurable prostate cancer, a disease he'll likely live with for several more years. She starts "There is a poem called 'Kindness' by Naomi Shihab Nye that stopped me in my tracks. It's one of the few things I ever memorized. It is so meaningful to me because I think it is kindness that I'm always trying to give to my husband, kindness that I am trying to give to myself, and kindness that I am trying to give to everybody else. The first few lines of the poem go like this:

Before you know what kindness really is
you must lose things,
feel the future dissolve in a moment
like salt in a weakened broth.

Her reflection on this poem completes the circle. "To know kindness you must lose things; we've all lost things, but we find things too."

Losing so that you may gain, giving away so that you may grow more rich, casting seeds out on to the ground so that they may come back a thousand fold—this is a biblical theme and an important theme in all of the world's great spiritual and wisdom traditions. Over and over on the weekend retreats, people show us how they face great losses with courage and faith and we watch as they grow to find greater peace and wisdom in their hearts. Feeling one's hopes, plans, and dreams of an imagined future dissolve "like salt in a weakened broth" is very painful, yet it also brings us a tenderness of heart that is loving kindness itself. Dissolving like salt in a weakened broth, we lose all that which keeps us small and separate, and we gain our true wholeness to merge with something bigger than ourselves, something universal, sacred, and holy.

CHAPTER 42

Continuing the Journey

Oh let me be an open-hearted man
Oh let me be an open hearted woman
Oh let me be the one who understands
Oh let me be the one who is filled with wisdom.
Words to song by Jason Schulman

Sunday afternoon. *We all gather in a large circle, holding hands and swaying back and forth, singing the final song of the weekend. There's an openness here where all emotions are welcome, and people look into each other's eyes uninhibited by shyness or preconception.*

The song finishes and a spontaneous 'hugfest' begins. The room is buzzing with conversation, heartfelt wishes, and the exchange of phone numbers and email addresses. People are soaking up the last few minutes. Slowly, in ones and twos they make their way to the door and back to their lives after the retreat.

What next?

At the end of the closing circle, we warn the group that healing can be a painful process. Like sitting on your foot while watching an engrossing movie, eventually you'll wake up to the fact that your foot is asleep. Awareness that you've neglected a part of yourself is the first painful step in reclaiming your already existing wholeness.

Likewise the emotional rawness many people experience at the end of a retreat takes time to heal. Hearing so many moving stories in such a short period takes time to digest and integrate into one's psyche. We encourage everyone to nurture their bodies with rest and healthy food, to make time for meditation and silence, and to mindfully connect with nature. All these self-care elements will help in the transition.

Many people will go home on such a high that they'll want to share the experience with their loved ones. We tell participants that we have heard that these conversations can fall flat because there's no way to capture in words the depth of love and peace experienced in the healing circle. We encourage them to be grateful and to settle for an inner smile of the heart. Their outward appearance may not change as they return to their families and the activities of living; people around them may not see or comprehend, at least initially, that they have been transformed.

Most people understand that the retreat represents a single step on their healing journey. Touched by the realm of spirit and possibility, participants resolve to direct loving-kindness towards their bodies, to practice mindfulness and the other healing skills, and to take additional steps to enrich their spiritual lives. But as is human, many will waver between actually following these aspirations and neglecting these healing practices.

They may watch themselves straying from a new healthy diet, or arguing with relatives, or letting their meditation practice slip. Old habits and the demands of their world will persist, and can quickly draw them back into the fray they wanted to avoid. Frustrations with themselves for regressing and worries that they're compromising their chance of recovery can continue to ebb and flow as they work to find their own rhythm of healing. Healing is a mysterious process, however, and its seed can be planted deep in the psyche and still grow.

Ordinary Yet Extraordinary People

The greatest power of the weekend retreat is in meeting ordinary yet extraordinary people who are travelling the same path. At a moment of despair, an image of someone who seemed to be struggling with the same issue and who was able to work through the tension, will pop into the mind. There will be a strong memory of a story of persistence, of holding a difficulty internally, then mixing that raw energy of emotion with wisdom and love, to create the fertile ground for transformation.

If a participant's motivation to stay on the healing journey wanes, sometimes he or she will remember the attributes of people who have beat all odds. Through spiritual practice, many of these remarkable survivors deliberately cultivated qualities that promoted their recovery. Beyond practising healing skills, these ordinary yet extraordinary people grappled with and resolved the most confusing paradoxes of life such as being able to accept their condition while actively promoting their health within and beyond the conventional medical system. Through deep struggles on the journey, they learned to cultivate a working trust in the innate healing power that comes from joining body, mind and spirit into an integral whole.

These remarkable people have also come to see the personal crisis of their cancer diagnosis as an opportunity for growth and personal transformation. Coming to see their cancer as a journey of the soul, they have learned not to see recurrence of cancer as a failure. Even in approaching death, they have found meaning and profound healing. Facing their fears, one by one, in the light of awareness has allowed them to let go of the armour around their heart to expose it again to the energies of life and the flow of love. In loving themselves, loving their families, friends and community, and allowing themselves to be loved, they have discovered that it is in igniting the wisdom fires of the heart that one is truly able to travel on the path of healing.

Your Transformation

The lessons of the retreat, and messages and images from reading this book, can resurface for you in the months and years to come. You are no different from the remarkable people you may read about. You have the capacity to empower yourself and truly make a difference in your health and all other aspects of your life.

There *is* a path towards complete healing but it takes practice and a willingness to stay with all the irritations, boredom, and pain that come on the spiritual journey. The instructions for the healing skills are here in this book. As you progress on your journey, you can trust in your innate wisdom and your yearning to heal to guide you to even further teachings.

Slowly, as if by grace, an internal transformation occurs. The early morning meditation practice begins to permeate the day. You may notice, even for brief moments, that time holds still. Awareness begins to grow, as you watch yourself breathing slowly and calmly into your belly, and as you allow your attention to hold your emotions and thoughts without getting caught up in them.

Mindfulness is no longer a concept, but a practice that opens the senses in moments of oneness, whether it is in looking at a flower or into the eyes of a loved one. More and more often, awareness shows the brilliance of everyday experiences. The world is the same, but somehow seems more vibrant, as if beautiful music was playing in the background. You, too, are the same but somehow transformed, able to appreciate the wholeness of your life, a wholeness that was there all along.

My Journey to Healing and Cancer
Timothy Walker

Compassion is not a relationship
between the healer and the wounded.
It's a relationship between equals.
Only when we know our own darkness well
can we be present with the darkness of others.
Compassion becomes real when
we recognize our shared humanity.
Pema Chrödrön

When Rob and I first met, I recognized early on that we were kindred spirits. He asked for meditation instruction, and as we started to meditate together, I felt connected with him in a deep stillness, presence and awareness. The space in the room became vivid and energized as inner chatter faded into a vast and open space of mind.

Back in the realm of our lively conversations, I found we also had a mutual vision and passion to bring the journey of personal development and spirituality into healthcare. Our friendship and collaboration since then has been a tremendous blessing in my life.

Over the years I have repeatedly been awestruck by Rob's commitment to personal growth, learning and awareness, both for himself and for others, as well as his tremendous discipline, energy and hard work. He has a unique skill in manifesting our vision by linking it to that of others so that it takes off like fire.

Ten years before that meeting with Rob, my mother had uterine cancer and I remember talking with her about some of the insights she derived from Bernie Siegel's book, *Love, Medicine and Miracles*, which she read while receiving her radiation treatments. Like many others, she was gutsy, proactive and determined to survive, for she had already been on a profound and difficult journey. Just a year before her diagnosis with cancer, she had been to detox and a twenty-eight day treatment program, for the second time in as many years. This second time it had "worked" and she was now an active and enthusiastic member of Alcoholics Anonymous. Her journey with this twelve step program brought her to spirituality and profound healing which she then brought directly into her experience with cancer.

In the many years preceding that, we didn't quite know why mom was so difficult and her behaviour so erratic. It wasn't until I was studying Systems Family Therapy, as part of my Masters Degree in Contemplative Psychotherapy, that it began to dawn on me that my mother was an alcoholic, just like her father had been, and that I had grown up in a distorted alcoholic family system. My father had been coming to me for years with his torment and concern for her, and I, as the dutiful son, was trying to help the best I could.

This family experience is perhaps part of why I became a seeker early in life, drawn to meditation, Buddhism, Yoga, Taoism, Mystical Christianity and Judaism, as well as poetry and Jungian depth psychology. I was looking for an answer to my confusion and self-created suffering.

In 1972, at age sixteen, I had been doing yoga and learned transcendental meditation, but did not find it truly satisfying. I kept seeking, reading mystical and Zen texts in undergraduate comparative religion classes and was inspired by the study of Chinese Philosophy.

It was only in 1979, when I first arrived at Naropa University (then Institute) as an aspiring and suffering poet, that I received formal instruction in Mindfulness Meditation within the Tibetan Buddhist Tradition. At that very moment, I knew I had found an immensely effective and profound way to work with my mind, emotions and suffering. I had found my genuine path toward wisdom, healing and awakening.

Daily meditation practice was bringing me insights into myself, and helping me to let go of the many years of accumulated patterns of confusion. The powerful relief I experienced led me to switch out of the poetry program at Naropa and into the Masters program in Contemplative Psychotherapy, thereby fully committing myself to the path of meditation and to the path of helping others.

This unique Masters program has as its most prominent feature a three-month retreat in the mountains of northern Colorado. It was this retreat that I was most yearning to experience. In retrospect, this retreat far exceeded my expectations and became the foundation of everything that I have done since.

Chögyam Trungpa Rinpoche, the famous Tibetan lama, was a pioneer in bringing Buddhism to the West and was the founder of Naropa University and Shambhala Buddhism. In the early seventies, he devised five meditation postures to be practiced in a set of five differently shaped and brightly coloured rooms. This practice, called Maitri Space Awareness, had the effect of heightening one's experience of both emotional energy and the potential wisdom or confusion that rises with that energy.

As part of the retreat, we trained in each of these rooms for a ten-day period, coupled with many hours of meditation and group process. The purpose was to derive insights into our unique personal patterns of confusion and then to liberate the energy and wisdom there with meditative awareness. Releasing patterns from the past, one finds a fresh and intelligent approach more relevant to the present moment. We also did a full month of traditional sitting meditation, ten hours a day, even eating our meals in a mindful style derived from Japanese Zen Buddhism.

I remember one day, near the end of the retreat, leaving the white room and walking alone across a snowy field. As I walked, my mind was completely still and focused in the present. I could feel my body in all its detail, in the richness and complexity of walking, breathing, and being. I could hear the crunch of snow under my feet and see the brightness of the sun glistening on the snow ahead. Then, as I crossed a little bridge and came up a small hill, I also had an extraordinary feeling of being at one with the environment. It was a feeling of being at one with the earth, the snow, the trees, the sky, and the universe, while also being a body that was walking in this environment. It felt to me as if this body, gently walking in the snow, was actually suspended from that greater space of mind, which was the environment, sky and universe beyond. As soon as I met one of my classmates further up the trail, the whole experience collapsed back into my normal discursive mode of being.

Upon leaving this retreat, I went straight into a one-year internship working in the mental health system. In the context of the training and experiences I'd had during the retreat and working with people who had severe mental illness, it became clear to me that we were all in the same boat. All of us were struggling with the same wild energies in our minds, bodies and emotions.

I realized that the confusion experienced by these people, who had been given the label of mental illness, and the confusion I experienced myself were fundamentally the same. The only difference was the intensity of their emotions and the persistence of their deluded states over long periods of time. I, too, had strong emotions and deluded states but I was learning, through meditation, to let go of fixed states of mind, to experience a gap and open to a natural, wakeful simplicity and sanity that was there in the mind all along.

Working with my mind and my emotions through meditation, I had learned that when I resist suffering, it festers and grows; and when I make friends with suffering, it softens and changes, eventually transforming altogether. I also learned to practice kindness and gentleness toward myself. Learning to open my heart to my own pain and struggles gave me the confidence to open my heart to the pain of others.

One young man I worked with, an artist and poet himself, felt tormented by demon voices one day and enticed by angelic visions the next. I spent many hours with him coming to understand the strange logic of his cosmology. At the same time, I also encouraged him to engage in ordinary activities with mindfulness, like doing his laundry and cleaning his room.

By attending to the details of simply being with him, without the concepts of diagnostic criteria or professional distance, it was easy to practice natural compassion. The word 'compassion', from the Latin, literally means to feel or suffer with another. My strong intention was to be with him so completely that I could ride with him through the depth of his pain and confusion with mental illness. As I relaxed into being with him, I seemed to resonate more and more with his experience, and I gradually made friends with the wild energies of his confusion and torment, as if they were my own.

After receiving my Masters degree, I worked for Naropa as a group leader and meditation instructor at two more of these three-month, Maitri Space Awareness, psychotherapy training retreats. I also participated in many other group and solo retreats over the next number of years.

During this period, I had the extreme privilege to be in the presence of and receive teachings from the Tibetan Lama and renowned meditation master Chögyam Trungpa Rinpoche. Beyond his vast learning both in the spiritual ways of the East and the West, he was also a poet and an artist, skilled in many different media. Perhaps what made him most unique, however, was his highly accomplished skill in that most difficult art, the art of being fully human.

As a young student with a deep desire to learn how to effectively help others, and with intense interest, I watched him as he taught, and especially the interactions he had with people during question and answer periods. He would hardly ever answer the words of the question directly but, instead, he would probe the person with his own questions to find out more about them and their life. Then he would guide them to their own insights. He would say something like "Well Sweetie, what do you think?" in his raspy high voice, putting the person on the spot so that they would blush, sweat and melt. With gentle skill and palpable compassion, he would awaken, within the questioner, their own inner wisdom that had long been sleeping. Through his presence, he seemed to guide people to be more truly present to the truth of who they are.

After finishing my Ph.D. in Halifax, Nova Scotia, I wanted to integrate meditation practice more into my counselling work. This desire led me to a professional training retreat with Dr. Jon Kabat-Zinn, another remarkable teacher who has successfully brought mindfulness meditation into the mainstream medical world. Being both a scientist and a seasoned meditation teacher, his published research and popular books on the effectiveness of mindfulness meditation in the context of stress reduction have allowed his model to spread to thousands of clinics and hospitals around the world.

I have deep respect and gratitude for Jon and what he has accomplished, for his tremendous generosity of spirit, and for his heartfelt dedication to the work of Mindfulness. I believe, one day, his work will be regarded as a major factor in creating a turning point in the history of healthcare. What I loved about training with Jon and love about teaching Mindfulness-Based Stress Reduction is how very practical the approach is, and how his language makes his approach relevant to everyone from all walks of life.

I opened my own Mindfulness-Based Stress Reduction Clinic early in 1996. It was within the next year that Rob gave me a call and we began to meet, to meditate together, and to talk about our passion for creating cancer support groups grounded in the ordinary spirituality of everyday life. I became very excited as we talked, especially when creating the curriculum for the first Skills for Healing Weekend Retreat.

I wanted to structure the program in such a way that we could create a very loving and safe environment for people to reach deep within themselves to find, what I tend to refer to as, their "golden heart of wisdom and compassion". I also wanted our program to go deeply into the root issues of peoples' suffering. I trusted that if people could thoroughly touch their suffering in the healing circle of love and awareness, then they would naturally awaken to the compassion and the wisdom of their healing heart. Over time, this principle has grown into what we call "going through the darkness to find the light" or, even more directly, "in the darkness is the light."

My inspiration, coming from the mindfulness meditation approach, is based in acknowledging that in life, cancer or no cancer, we all share a fundamental common experience of suffering, of stress, of resistance to change, of a struggle in our lives to grow and learn. We all share the fear of sickness and the fear of death and the fear of losing loved ones. I wanted to create an opportunity for people to heal into wholeness. Wholeness comes about when we integrate body, emotions, mind and spirit and when we open our hearts to others in our family, community and the world.

Most of us in our current society live lives fractured into many different pieces that we put into different compartments. We also tend to armour our hearts against loss, pain and suffering. When a cancer diagnosis occurs for ourselves or our loved ones, a further shattering occurs as many of the normal reference points, we have come to rely on, start to fall apart.

When a shattering occurs in our life, it is an invitation to seek a greater wholeness beyond this shattering. I have had the privilege to study for the last 12 years with Jason Shulman, a master healer, Buddhist and Kabbalah teacher, who has taught me that in my own shattering I can release into an already existing wholeness. This already existing wholeness has no boundaries and therefore cannot be shattered but can hold all the shattering of the world. He has taught me to honour the shattering as a necessary part of awakening to this greater wholeness. He has created a powerful system of healing, Integrated Kabbalistic Healing, based on the tree of life in the mystical teachings of Judaism.

At the heart of this system are the principles of relationship and integration. Healing occurs in relationship and healing brings integration. When we open our hearts to share our deepest pain and fear with others, when we acknowledge honestly, in relationship, where and how our life is shattered, we begin to ignite the fires of compassion in our hearts and in the hearts of others.

This holy fire of love and compassion forms connections between people and within ourselves, connecting body, emotions, mind and spirit into a fluid and integrated whole. When we glimpse this greater wholeness, our shattering is held in a bigger space of awareness with tender, loving kindness, allowing us to breathe with a soft belly and feel the richness of life with a tender open heart.

All of these principles were essential to the structure and curriculum of our weekend retreats for people with cancer; trusting in the already existing wholeness and the heart of wisdom and compassion; knowing that in the darkness is the light; and believing that when body, emotions, mind and spirit flow together and integrate, then people begin to heal.

Our retreats invited people to bring whatever was present for them in their current states: all of their feelings, all their problems, all of their fears, and all their concerns, as well as the richness of their stories of humour and triumph, of joy and inspiration.

As people slowly filed into the large old ballroom of a former nurses' residence for the first Skills for Healing Weekend retreat in November 1999, as they took their seats in the big circle of chairs, I think Rob and I were both floating three feet off the ground, nerves tingling with excitement, fear and anticipation. After we made our introductory statements, a hush fell over the room. Then, when Rob invited people to tell their cancer story and to speak from their heart about what they had found most difficult, the magic truly began.

From that day to this, we have both been deeply moved, and at times awe-struck, by the courage, strength, resiliency and love expressed by these people who have faced cancer and shared their stories of life and healing in the healing circle with strangers. My aspiration now is to expand this healing circle to include as many people as possible and to continue deepening the work by creating longer retreats where people can further develop their shining hearts of wisdom, compassion and the power to heal.

Acknowledgements from Rob and Tim

For nearly three years, we have spent many nights and weekends together hunched over a laptop, sometimes wiping away tears while writing, reading and editing the powerful stories you will find in this book. Our friendship in spirit, sustained by our love for facilitating retreats, has been cured in the fire of learning from each other and writing this together. Our mutual respect and gratitude for one another is truly a blessing.

We also feel a vast sense of gratitude for all the other people who have been a part of the web of exertion, stories, and wisdom that have made this book and the Healing and Cancer Foundation a reality. Contemplating all the people who have enabled us is overwhelming. We are afraid these words cannot convey the deep sense of appreciation and love we feel for all of the people who have given so much.

Sitting on the Shoulders of Giants

We would like to acknowledge all the pioneers who have come before us, blazing the trail of establishing and running cancer support groups. Dr. David Spiegel, Dr. Irving Yalom, and, of course, Dr. Bernie Siegel, who inspired Rob to become an oncologist. Special among these is our friend and mentor, Dr. Alastair Cunningham, who pioneered the Healing Journey Program at the Princess Margaret hospital in Toronto for the past 25 years. He has been a tireless advocate for bringing spirituality and healing into modern medicine and offered valuable feedback on the manuscript.

In particular, Tim was fortunate to study and train with many exceptional teachers. Chief among these is the Tibetan meditation master Chogyam Trungpa Rinpoche whose transformative presence, compassion and wisdom have echoed in the retreats and resonates in the writing of this book. The Shambhala teachings of Sakyong Mipham Rinpoche have continued this legacy. At Naropa, Tim also met the great Christian contemplatives; Father Thomas Keating, Brother David Stiendl-Rast, Father William MacNamaera, and Mother Tessa Bielecki who helped him see the jewel of the spiritual life from different angles. Pema Chrodron's kind presence and many books inspired Tim, while Dr. Ed Podvol and

Jeff Fortuna first taught him the power of healing circles. Alan Ginsburg transmitted the sacred power of language and Jon Kabbat-Zinn truly gave a gift that has multiplied a thousand fold. Tim's Dharma brother, healer and Kabbalah teacher, Jason Shulman, taught reclaiming wholeness for self and others.

Rob especially feels honoured to be part of the medical system and its age-old tradition of apprenticeship and the principle of dedicating one's life in the service of others. His professors and teachers in medical school in Toronto, and mentor Radiation Oncologists in Ottawa, will always remain as nurturing parents in his psyche. He notes that the social workers, Gill Reilly, Susan Kenney, and Sydney Foran should be recognized for the amazing work they do daily, and for having the courage to take a young resident/radiation oncologist interested in support groups under their wings.

The Wise Editors

In preparing our manuscript, we have also been blessed along the way with wise counsel. Emily Sell got us started, helping us to shape our ideas, to make the leap from spoken lectures to literary art, and to understand the crucial lesson, "Show, don't tell." Paul Halpern made our first draft respectable with his keen eye for detail, while he himself was struggling with the cancer that took his life in the fall of 2008. He was a warrior of the spirit and is greatly missed. Finally our collaboration with Liz Crocker in the final months has been a joy. She jumped into the project in midstream, to do the lion's share of the editing, out of the kindness of her heart and the motivation to empower people seeking medical care. Her lifetime of loving books and people and her lived wisdom are reflected beautifully in many elements of our book. Our book designer, Kathy Kaulbach, seemed to appear just when we needed her most.

The Healing and Cancer Foundation

What began as a dream shared together while driving or flying back home from teaching retreats, in our excited conversations and fond memories of wise characters, went from scribbled notes to this book because of the fabulous friendship and immense talents of Boyd Sharpe. Boyd, supported by his wife Juanita, has become our indispensable audio, video, website, techno-wizard without whom all of this would have been lost, forgotten in our Monday morning clinic-minds. Boyd has also become a founding member on the Healing and Cancer Foundation board along with Rita Thompson and Kathy McLaughlin.

Rita and Kathy have been instrumental in helping us take teachings from the weekend retreats and turn them into a charitable organization which will freely share our experience with countless others. As well, Kathy's chapter (Miracles can Happen) emerged from her own writing to become part of this book, and Rita gave her inscrutable critic's eye to line edit and proof read at various stages of the manuscript. Rita has also offered sage advice at every step along the way on business and legal matters, while Kathy's executive coaching experience, facilitation skills and marketing knowledge have kept our progress on track. Many other people have helped our Foundation, like the volunteer transcriptionists, and we feel blessed with all their hard work and passion for our projects.

Retreat Organizers

Huge thanks go to all of the local organizers of the 26 weekend retreats, in fifteen cities, over the last decade. The retreats would not happen without these volunteers stepping forward to get the word out, find a venue, set up a registration system, order catering, make photocopies, collate evaluations and all of the other tasks, great and small, that go into mounting a retreat.

We are grateful to the many volunteer facilitators who added their healing presence and expertise in leading small groups. Our gratitude also goes out to the financial sponsors of the retreats: multiple pharmaceutical companies (Abbott, Astrazeneca, Novartis, OrthoBiotech, Paladin, Perdue, Pfizer, Roche, Sanofi-Aventis, Schering); and various organizations like the Canadian Cancer Society, Wellspring, HopeSpring, HearthPlace, several Regional Cancer Centres, and many more.

The Stars of the Stories

Most importantly, we are deeply grateful to all of the participants of our Skills for Healing Weekend Retreats over the last ten years. They have taught us and enriched our lives immeasurably. Their stories truly make this book come alive.

Willing to gather in the healing circle with strangers, they quickly learned to appreciate one another for all their quirkiness, grit, humour and intelligence. They demonstrated such bravery, with all of their vulnerability, tenderness, tears and confused emotions, as they faced their greatest fears and found within themselves a deeply abiding strength and wisdom for healing. They demonstrated, in retreat after retreat, the resilience of the human spirit. It has been beautiful to witness.

It is important to note that each of the story chapters represents only a tiny sliver of much richer lives. We wish you could know each of them as we do and we thank them all.

Andrew is a writer and a humorist. He generously offered up his own writing to use in this book. It would not be fair to thank Andrew without also acknowledging his wonderful wife, Velma, who was patiently opening his mind long before his awake craniotomy.

Marie was the first person who was videotaped and gave her story with enthusiasm and heartfulness.

Karen demonstrated tremendous courage in her willingness to face the darkness completely and come out the other side.

Geoff, a remarkable young leader and visionary, has become a dear friend and collaborated with us for two years to create retreats for his organization Young Adult Cancer Canada.

Bonnie, the spirited kayaker, sent us emails and talked with us on the phone to fill in her story. She continues to enrich our lives.

Cathy generously gave us her story about coming back from the brink of death a changed woman.

Pam had such a commanding presence in the small groups, spellbinding those who listened to her, as she generously gave her story after all the struggles in her life.

Jackie's two stories have brought tears to our eyes with every reading. She had a deep commitment to spiritual growth and we miss her boisterous laugh and her refreshing honesty.

Harry, our Santa Claus friend, discovered, beyond all expectations, that he actually liked meditating! We are grateful he has offered his story of his wife, Ann, who participated so fully in the retreat despite her advanced stage of carcinoid cancer.

Peter, whose heart is big enough to be a lumberjack and a nurse, and Janet whose spirit shines, God Bless you both.

Christine clarified many points with us in several conversations and offered so much of herself in the small groups as well as in interviews and emails. We are grateful that her story includes some of her experiences with Alix, a very gifted spiritual healer who was, like Tim, also a student of Jason Shulman's and an esteemed teacher in his school. Alix's healing presence is greatly missed by many.

Julie has told her story on multiple occasions and every time we have been deeply moved. She also agreed to be videotaped and star in her own story which you can watch at www.HealingandCancer.org. Her story also includes Randy's story, a great cancer warrior to whom we are also eternally grateful.

Special Words from Timothy Walker, PhD.

Though my family and friends have often missed me while writing, their love is steadfast and their support essential. Thanks especially to Erin, Sophia, Annie, Dorothy and to the cradling matrix of my beloved community.

Heartfelt Thanks from Dr. Rob Rutledge

To the people I work with everyday, Marsha Avery, Dorreen Westhaver, the radiation therapists, nurses, and all the staff at the cancer centre: you are angels in this world. I am also indebted to my colleagues, and the Head of Radiation Oncology, Dr. Tetteh Ago, for supporting me and allowing me to facilitate support groups, and to speak and write about my passion. Thank you all for accepting me for who I am.

I also want to acknowledge that this book would not have come to life without the endless support my wife, Cara, and the understanding and patience of our two sons, Jeremy and Graham. Their love is the food for my soul.

Suggested Reading

Anti-Cancer: A New Way of Life
David Servan-Schreiber (2007). Collins: Toronto, ON

This is a compelling story of Dr. Servan-Schreiber, a psychiatrist and neuroscientist, who developed brain tumour, had surgery, and then experienced a recurrence of his cancer. Based on both the insights he gained through his cancer journey and his research into the causes of cancer, Dr. Servan-Schreiber integrates the scientific explanation of genetics, diet, psycho-neuro-immunology, and mind-body medicine with practical advice and common-sense wisdom to support our natural capacity for healing. A removable guide called "Anticancer Action" is included at the end of the book. While 'cancer' is in the title, it translates to all areas of health.

Fighting Cancer from Within: How to Use the Power of Your Mind for Healing
Martin L. Rossman M.D. (2003). Henry Holt & Co.: New York, NY

Presented as a compliment to standard medical practices, this is a comprehensive guide to using imagery throughout the different phases of the cancer experience. The book provides cancer patients with imagery techniques designed to reduce the stress of their initial shock at the time of diagnosis; methods which can facilitate healing from surgery and enhance immune function; approaches to help tolerate the side-effects of chemotherapy and radiation; and perspectives on ways to foster the journey of healing and recovery. A set of guided imagery CDs is also available.

Full Catastrophe Living: Using the Wisdom of Your Body and Mind to Face Stress, Pain and Illness
Jon Kabat-Zinn, Ph.D. (1990) Random House: New York, NY

Jon Kabat-Zinn founded the Mindfulness-Based Stress Reduction Clinic at the University of Massachusetts Medical Center. By describing what goes on at this Clinic, Jon manages to weave together sound science, rich stories, and profound teachings on meditation as a path toward healing and wholeness. Filled with practical guidance for everyday life as well as for extreme states of pain, illness and anxiety, this book is a true and wise resource worthy of being read again and again. Having stood the test of time, *Full Catastrophe Living* has become a classic. (Other recommended books by Jon Kabat-Zinn: *Wherever You Go, There You Are* and *Coming To Our Senses).*

Kitchen Table Wisdom: Stories that Heal
Rachel Naomi Remen, M.D. (1996). Riverhead Books: New York, NY

This is a remarkable collection of true stories from the 'kitchen table' tradition of shared human experience, showing us life in all its power and mystery. Remen believes in the power of stories and says "Facts bring us to knowledge but stories bring us to wisdom." She skilfully includes her own story of awakening to wisdom and healing in her own life as a paediatrician and Professor of Medicine. Through her own story and stories of her patients, she shows this wisdom has existed all along, underneath the routines of medical technology and medical personae. Every story, layered with beautiful metaphors, has profound lessons to teach all of us and merits multiple readings.

Love, Medicine and Miracles: Lessons Learned about Self-Healing from a Surgeon's Experience with Exceptional Patients
Bernie Siegel, M.D., (1986). Quill Publishing: Minneapolis, MN

The cover description of this classic book written by a cancer surgeon beautifully captures its essence: "Unconditional love is the most powerful stimulant of the immune system. The truth is: love heals. Miracles happen to exceptional patients every day--patients who have the courage to love, those who have the courage to work with their doctors to participate in and influence their own recovery". *(This book inspired Rob Rutledge to become an oncologist and run cancer support groups.)*

Loving Kindness: The Revolutionary Art of Happiness
Sharon Salzberg (1995) Shambhala Publications: Boston, MA

This book gives detailed instructions on how to practice loving kindness meditation and provides excellent examples and stories about how loving kindness can make a difference in your everyday life. These profound teachings, when taken to heart and practiced, help you to appreciate not only the beautiful mystery of life but also other people, whether close friends and family, those you struggle to accept, or even those you have never met. The healing power of these practices occurs on many layers of your life.

Picking up the Pieces: Moving Forward After a Cancer Diagnosis
Sherri Magee, PhD. (2006). Raincoast Books: Vancouver, BC.

Practical, reassuring and informative, *Picking Up the Pieces* is based on four years of research and interviews with hundreds of people who have lived through a cancer diagnosis. Dr. Magee guides survivors through a unique process, including daily practices, that builds a bridge from hospital to home, and beyond. The book's deep psychological and spiritual explorations are rarely presented with such warmth and insight.

Privileged Presence: Personal Stories of Connections in Health Care
Liz Crocker & Bev Johnson (2006). Bull Publishing Company: Boulder, CO

This book is a collection of more than 50 true stories from the points of view of patients, family members and health care professionals. They share the wisdom that has come from personal experiences in a wide range of health care situations and settings. At their core, the stories are all about how people connect with others, or miss the opportunity to connect, and the difference that makes. Some stories will warm your heart and some will make your jaw drop, but they all
contain insights about how people want to be treated with respect and dignity; with compassion; with open communication; and in a spirit of a full collaborative partnership.

The Art of Emotional Healing
Lucia Capacchione (2001). Shambhala Publications: Boston, MA

This book offers a rich array of tools, ideas, exercises, experiences and wisdom to help you work through emotional turmoil to add tremendous richness and colour to your life. Topics include learning to experience emotions as energy; how emotions get stored in our body; and discovering the art of emotional expression with many different creative media, including visual arts, sculpture, masks, sound, writing, dialoguing, dance and storytelling. This is an excellent guide for anyone who wants to explore the unfolding mystery of their inner life through experiencing artistic expression.

The Healing Journey: Overcoming the Crisis of Cancer
Alastair J. Cunningham (1992, 2000). Key Porter Books: Toronto, ON

Dr. Alastair Cunningham is a scientist, psychologist, and cancer survivor himself. He presents a balanced survey of self-help approaches with the aim of helping you plan your own healing journey. He explains, in lay terms, conventional medical approaches, dietary remedies, psychological interventions, and spiritual perspectives that can be helpful to those with cancer. Dr. Cunningham founded, and directed for 25 years, the Healing Journey program at the Princess Margaret Hospital (PMH), in Toronto, Canada. Visit www.healingjourney.ca to learn more.

The Places That Scare You: a Guide to Fearlessness in Difficult Times
Pema Chrödrön (2001). Shambhala: Boston, MA

"We can let the circumstances of our lives harden us and make us increasingly resentful and afraid, or we can let them soften us and make us kinder and more open to what scares us. We always have this choice." With this, Pema Chrödrön, an American Grandmother and Buddhist Nun, begins her teachings on developing a tender heart that contains both courage and compassion. Applicable to everyone, Pema's writing is pithy, insightful, warm-hearted and profound. *The Places that Scare You* is filled with stories and examples that speak to universal human themes. Pema has written many other books, all of which are recommended.

Turning The Mind Into An Ally
Sakyong Mipham (2003). Riverhead Books: New York

This is an essential read for anyone who is interested in establishing, deepening and maintaining a consistent meditation practice. The author, a master of meditation, often uses the analogy of meditation as riding a wild horse. He guides the reader, step by step, to train one's mind in stability, clarity and strength to eventually develop awareness, insight and wisdom. With simple, fresh language and engaging examples, he shows us that "true happiness is always available to us, but first we have to create the environment for it to flourish".

The Power Of Now: A Guide to Spiritual Enlightenment
Eckhart Tolle (1997). Namaste Publishing: Vancouver, BC

Even while reading this extraordinary book, you can begin to feel the difference of awakening to the 'Now'. Tolle presents rational and clear arguments to explain that time is a delusion, that all problems are illusions of the mind, that the loss of 'now' is the core delusion, and that we can transform illness into enlightenment and suffering into peace. Tolle's own personal enlightenment erupted out of tremendous confusion and pain. He eloquently describes how you too can bring about a similar shift in your consciousness. Other books by Ekhart Tolle are also highly recommended.

Agenda of a "Skills For Healing" Weekend Retreat

Friday Evening • Empowering the Body

5:30   Introduction
Drs. Rob Rutledge and Timothy Walker share their stories and the overview of the retreat.

6:00   Opening circle
Each attendee is asked to share what has been most difficult on their cancer journey and their hopes for the weekend.

7:30   Lecture: Complete Cancer Care
Rob outlines how to get the best medical care with other ways to empower body, mind and spirit.

8:15   Introduction to Meditation
Tim starts by focusing on body, breath and the feeling of being alive.

Saturday Morning • Settling the Mind

9:00   Mediation: Thoughts are Like Clouds

9:15   Introduction to Mindfulness
Tim explains the power of bringing your attention into the here and now.

9:30   Raisin Eating Meditation
Each person eats a raisin slowly and mindfully to experience how they might also taste the true richness of their life in every moment.

9:45   Relaxation Breath and Body Scan
Tim teaches how to tap into the relaxation response through breath and mindful attention to each part of the body in turn.

11:00   Lecture: Stress and the Relaxation Response
Rob reviews the physiology of stress and burnout.

11:30   Small Group Discussion on Stress
Each person identifies stressors, their own stress reactions, and ways they help themselves.

Saturday Afternoon • Reframing Distressing Thoughts

1:30   Qi Gong
A gentle and easy standing exercise, this ancient Chinese practice helps refresh one's 'chi'.

2:00   Lecture: Reframing Distressing Thoughts with Wisdom and Kindness
This three-step approach shows how to work with difficult thoughts and emotions.

2:45   Small Group Discussion on Reframing Distressing Thoughts
Each person works with their own distressing thoughts to find a wise and kind 'reframe'.

4:00   Meditation: Alchemy of the Heart

Sunday Morning • Reclaiming our Wholeness

9:00   Meditation: Bowl of Loving Kindness
Everyone imagines that they could pour all their love as well as their 'negative' emotions into a bowl, allowing the energies to mix and the difficulties to be transformed.

9:15   Talk: Fears and Hopes
Tim illustrates, both personally and generally, how embracing fear can liberate life.

9:45   Small Group Discussion on Fears and Hopes
Each person shares their greatest fears, how their priorities have changed since the cancer diagnosis, and their hopes for the future.

11:00   Yoga
This gentle exercise, done while lying on mats, finishes with a 'rain of healing' visualization.

11:45   Talk: Spirituality and wholeness
This secular approach to spirituality offers a variety of approaches to access and experience the sacred in everyday life.

1:30   Closing Circle
Each person shares their insights and reflections from the weekend retreat.

Please visit *HealingandCancer.org* to learn more about upcoming retreats and other events or to freely view all the retreat lectures and discussions.